ZIEGFELD GIRL

ZIEGFELD GIRL

Image and

Icon in Culture

and Cinema

Linda Mizejewski

Duke University Press

Durham & London

1999

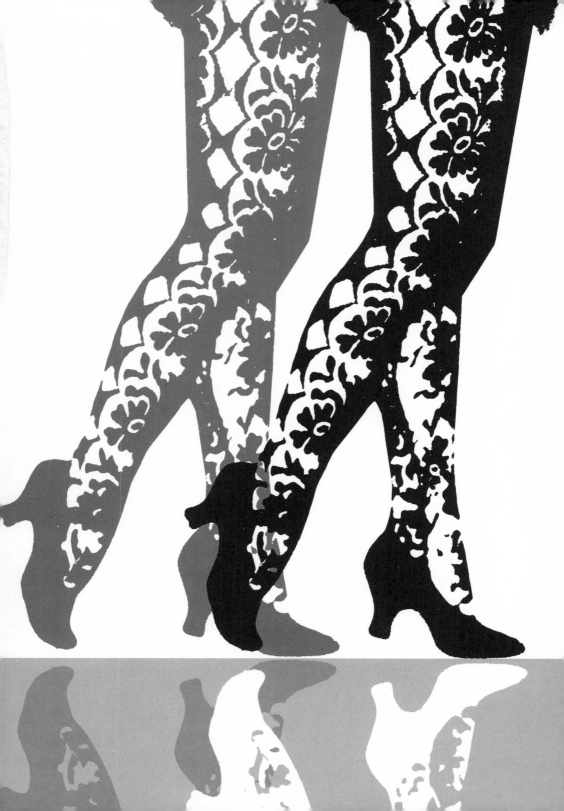

© 1999 Duke University Press

All rights reserved

Printed in the United States of America on acid-free paper ∞

Typeset in Dante with Bremen and

Monoline Script display by Tseng Information Systems, Inc.

Library of Congress Cataloging-in-Publication Data

appear on the last printed page of this book.

for George Cowmeadow Bauman

CONTENTS

ACKNOWLEDGMENTS

A rich network of personal and institutional support made it possible for me to complete this book. I am truly indebted to my friends and colleagues Judith Mayne and Debra Moddelmog, who patiently read versions of the entire manuscript and unfailingly gave me excellent advice. My thanks also goes to Peter Bailey, Lewis A. Erenberg, Ruth Lindeborg, and the readers at Duke University Press for helpful suggestions and recommendations. I owe a great deal to Pamela Brown for sharing her work on Anna Held and for influencing my thoughts about this celebrity. Elizabeth Taylor, Susan Essman, Stacey Klein, and Jill Jones-Renger, my research assistants at Ohio State University, all deserve credit for their meticulous work and reliability.

Very early in this project, Lucy Fischer, Dana Polan, Marcia Landy, and James Knapp at the University of Pittsburgh offered encouragement and insights. Thanks also goes to my colleagues in the English Department at Ohio State who have cheerfully listened to my papers and ideas about Ziegfeld Girls over the past years with interest and good questions. In the final stages of this project, I have appreciated the promptness, courtesy, and professional guidance of Ken Wissoker at Duke University Press.

Fellowships from the American Council of Learned Societies and the National Endowment for Humanities enabled me to complete my research and draft this manuscript. Grants-in-aid from the College of Humanities and the Office of Research and Graduate Studies at Ohio State University provided further funding for research and materials. I have been fortunate to have the support of Morris Beja and James Phelan, consecutive chairs of the English Department at Ohio State, who consistently endorsed my requests for time and assistance.

My thanks also goes to the staffs of the Billy Rose Theatre Collection, New York Public Library for the Performing Arts; the Curtis Theater Collection, University of Pittsburgh; and the Theater Arts Collection, Harry Ransom Humanities Research Center, University of Texas at Austin. At the latter, Melissa Miller was particularly thoughtful and generous with her help.

As the paragraphs above suggest, many privileges make this kind of research work possible. I am fortunate to have friends who helped me see this bigger picture on my more myopic days. Debra Bruce, Elizabeth Coffman, Karen Ford, Ursula Ganz-Blaettler, Rose Gatens, Meg Geroch, Tom Jeffers, Rita Mayer, Charlotte Mears, Ann Molnar, Jan and Fran Polek, Carolyn Rhodes, Jerzyna Slomczynska, Dick Thomas, and Jean Wyatt offered comfort, coffee, lecture opportunities, or sounding boards at crucial moments. For unwavering confidence and excitement about my work, I could always count on my family: my parents, sisters, and brothers, particularly my mother, who should have been a Ziegfeld Girl, and my brother Edward Vargas, who entertained me with stories about movies and showgirls before I knew how to read. I am most of all grateful to George Cowmeadow Bauman, whose care, affection, and enthusiasm carried me through this project.

INTRODUCTION

Glory, Legend, and the Ziegfeld Guarantee

Through most of the twentieth century, American popular culture has staged some incarnation of the Ziegfeld Girl, often in her trademark six-foot feather headdresses, parading and posing, occasionally singing and dancing, or floating down staircases and ramps, demonstrating the haughty Ziegfeld Walk. American theater's most enduring showgirl was the Follies Girl from Florenz Ziegfeld Jr.'s renowned revues, which ran on Broadway from 1907 to 1931. In the decades after she disappeared from the stage, versions of Ziegfeld's showgirl haunted musical films paying direct or indirect homage to the entrepid producer and his glorious Girl. Choreographer Busby Berkeley, who apprenticed with Ziegfeld late in the latter's career, endlessly duplicated Ziegfeldesque showgirls in musicals of the 1930s and 1940s. Metro Goldwyn Mayer (MGM) produced a lavish musical tribute in Robert Z. Leonard's *The Great Ziegfeld* in 1936 and even attempted to re-create the original Broadway revue in *The Ziegfeld Follies* film ten years later. Leonard's 1941 film *Ziegfeld Girl* emblazoned the brand name in popular culture, replacing the "Follies Girl" moniker with one more directly associated with the eminent producer. The name by then was shorthand for glory and glamour: Ziegfeld stars, the Ziegfeld stage, Ziegfeld Girls.

More recently, Ziegfeld Girls have reappeared on Broadway as characters in *Ziegfeld: A Night at the Follies* (1989) and in the long-running *Will Rogers Follies* (1991). In campier versions, they were crystallized into drag queens off-Broadway in Howard Crabtree's 1993 *Whoop-Dee-Doo!* and into retro burlesque figures in Madonna's touring *Girlie Show* the same year. An older generation may remember Ziegfeld showgirls such as Marilyn Miller, and theater buffs may recognize the names of Lillian Lorraine and Gilda Gray. But the Ziegfeld Girl today is probably best known through her fictional counterparts and allusions, such as the movie characterizations by Lana Turner and Hedy Lamarr, and the tributes of Madonna and off-Broadway men in drag.

Endlessly promoted by the Ziegfeld office and later lionized by the popular press, the Ziegfeld Girl has likewise acquired a weighty history in trade and tabloid publications, Broadway chronicles, and feature-story journalism. In the late 1990s, as promoters attempt to straighten Times Square into a Disney-safe family space, the Ziegfeld Girl still occasionally surfaces in newspaper and magazine articles lamenting the demise of the naughty grand old revue days. The tone of these references often hovers delicately between reverence and camp. A 1996 *New York Times* article described the Ziegfeld Girls as "legendary" inhabitants of "glory days" and a "fairy-tale world," as "glorious specimens of American womanhood" who "were choreographed to convey desire." In 1997, the *London Times* included Florenz Ziegfeld as one of history's most important musical producers, yet it featured a photograph not of his many musical stars but of a bevy of 1920s Follies Girls with the caption, "Glory days: Florenz Ziegfeld said his *Follies* were designed to glorify the American Girl."[1]

The Glorified American Girl became the *Follies'* official theme and rubric in 1922. However, nationalist rhetoric, the suggestion that there was something specifically "American" about the highly select Follies Girls, had flavored Ziegfeld publicity for the previous eight years. The rhetoric was well suited to revue-style patriotism, which was evident even earlier in Ziegfeld's grand production pieces. Follies Girls wore battleship headdresses to salute the U.S. Navy in 1909, and in other numbers throughout the years, they posed as Fourth of July sparklers, minutemen, or as more lofty figures of democracy and sacrifice during the Great War. Describing a *Follies* rendition of the national anthem, a 1915 reviewer noted that "not since Perry's men stripped and fought naked aboard the 'Lawrence' has there been so much undressing on behalf of this sweet land of liberty."[2] American expansionism and foreign interests similarly provided occasions for revue extravaganzas; in the 1913 *Follies*, Ziegfeld Girls "swam" in the background as a Ziegfeld remake of the Panama Canal opened center stage.

Other American desires were played out and put on display as well. Rapidly developing consumerism merged seamlessly with over-the-top revue style; in some of their best-known production numbers, Ziegfeld showgirls formed lines of Cartier jewelry, posed as fashion accessories and brand-name drinks, and were arranged in tableaux of the grand tour

and the society wedding. When Ziegfeld began to hire fashion mannequins as showgirls in 1915, his pageants functioned even more literally as
upscale department store windows featuring influential models of products, consumption, and bodies.

The Ziegfeld public relations office regularly announced the high cost
and authenticity of the jewels, fabrics, and furs onstage, implying the superior quality of the Girls as well. Most journalists and reviewers of the
era eagerly participated in the rhetoric of a guarantee of quality. "Trademarking chorus girls is one of the best things Florenz Ziegfeld does,"
claimed a 1915 newspaper article. "Once Flo sizes up a girl, accepts her
and puts her in a Follie or a Frolic, that girl bears forever a hallmark
just as plainly as though a device were stamped upon her lovely arm." [3]
Contemporary readers may wince at the latter-day connotations of a
tattoo. The more pertinent analog may be the Universal Product Code,
but categorization and brand-name recognition in fact characterize the
Ziegfeld Girl as much as her regulation feathers and headdress.

In 1929, Alexander Woollcott assessed Ziegfeld's advertising tactics
with a mixture of irony and genuine admiration, pointing out that the
Ziegfeld name had become "a trade-mark, a kind of universal guarantee"
for "more squanderous settings, lovelier pageantry, and damsels fairer to
see than you would find on any other stage in the land." [4] Eventually, the
rhetoric and publicity of Ziegfeld's *Follies* focused on nationalist themes
around the Follies Girls themselves, describing them as "strictly American" and claiming for them an authenticity of nationality to match the
authenticity of the silks and pearls onstage. The "universal guarantee" of
Ziegfeld's trademark showgirl entailed not just looks and costumes but
also a race and class identification as desirable, marketable, and genuinely American.

My own interest and the topic of this book is the Ziegfeld showgirl's
embodiment of this larger category or fantasy of American womanhood,
at once a fluffy publicity gimmick and an enduring assumption casually invoked by the *New York Times* nearly a century later. My premise
is that the Ziegfeld Girl in her many images—fashion model, showgirl,
Glorified American Girl—worked as a powerful icon of race, sexuality,
class, and consumerist desires early in this century, with resonances
persisting into the present day. As an icon, this figure continues to be

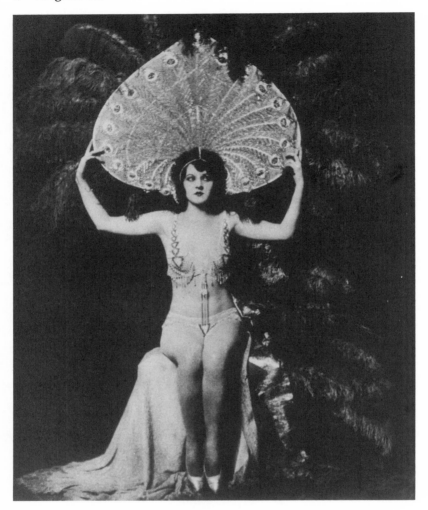

The Ziegfeld Girl as "guarantee" of body and costume: Katherine Burke in the *Follies,* circa 1928.

reproduced as the site of legends, stories, and interpretations of a social era.[5] Thousands of women were Ziegfeld Girls, real historical subjects, about whom much has been written as biography and theater history. This book supplements and questions that history by focusing on the Ziegfeld Girl's meanings as a "trademark" and identity.

Regarding this iconography, my assumption is that the Ziegfeld Girl was not only a signifier of urgent social issues but was also herself an important site of these issues, an example of how the body itself operates as the material of history. While her status as an icon maps out her circulation through American culture, her status as a particular, disciplined body situates the Ziegfeld Girl as one specific terrain of that culture. In a history of sexuality, she powerfully illustrates how such a history is materialized through racial, ethnic, economic, and nationalist contentions.

In the first decades of this century, Broadway teemed with show-girls and brand-name revue girls, but the Ziegfeld Girl's afterlife has remained unique in its scope, variety, and perpetuity. In addition, she has generated multiple interpretations and uses, crisscrossing American popular culture as legend, nostalgia, and camp. Thus she has been identified as fashion icon, modern glamour, national symbol, and image of the Roaring Twenties, but also as a rich resource of gay humor, as evidenced in the Ziegfeldesque revue *Whoop-Dee-Doo!* The excessiveness of her plumage and poses threatens to expose sex and gender distinctions as matters of costume and lighting. The drop-dead earnestness of Ziegfeld Girl pageantry likewise tips even her most serious representations into camp: in *Ziegfeld Girl*, Lana Turner lies dying in the lobby while Judy Garland triumphs on top of a giant wedding cake made of other Ziegfeld Girls; in *Broadway Melody* (Harry Beaumont, 1929), the lucky gal chosen for stardom by "the Great Zanfield" poses motionless in spangled undies in a Roman Empire tableau.

The reversibility as well as the specific gender and cultural stakes of the Ziegfeld Girl's meanings are suggested in William Wyler's 1968 film *Funny Girl*. Barbra Streisand as Fanny Brice exclaims, upon her discovery and ordination by the great producer, "I'm a Ziegfeld Girl!" At least in this version of Brice's life, however, the singer knows immediately that in spite of her talents, she is vastly different from the showgirl-variety Ziegfeld Girls. Ziegfeld includes her in the show's grand bridal finale because, he says, he needs "a strong voice," but Brice reads the song lyrics and quickly realizes she does not have the matching body and face for a number about wedding-day beauty. Instead, Brice tucks a pillow under her skirt and steals the scene as a clowning, very pregnant bride, an earthy, outrageous contrast to the ethereal Ziegfeld Girls

floating around her. The pregnant bride satirizes the real distance between biology and the Ziegfeld Girl's untouchable, mannequin-perfect
chic. More than that, pregnancy and comedy in tandem summarize a
transgressive, out-of-male-control power wholly verboten in disciplined
Ziegfeld Girlhood. As the film makes clear, Brice's comic genius was her
embodiment of everything the Ziegfeld Girl was forbidden to be: spon-
taneous, loud, clumsy, ethnic, Jewish.

Top-notch comedians such as Fanny Brice were a staple of Ziegfeld's *Follies* but were publicized and featured differently from the leggy,
ornately costumed Girls. The revue structure alternated full-stage pageant numbers with musical and comedy routines. The rhythm of the
revue depended on the juxtaposition of the sparkling, extended spectacle scenes with the snappy variety numbers in between. Whereas the
showgirl spectacles slowed down the pace for a more leisurely feast for
the eyes, the revue moved along quickly, with simpler and smaller performances staged to keep the audience busy while elaborate stagings
were set up behind the curtains.

The Follies Girls sometimes posed as background or provided chorus
support for the other acts, but they were the raison d'être and the center-
pieces of the grand parade and tableau productions. In the renowned
"living curtain" effect of Ziegfeld pageantry, female bodies were literally
conflated into the dazzling mise-en-scène. These showstopping, full-
stage numbers quickly became the hallmark of Ziegfeld's shows. Anecdotes about the *Follies* often suggested that the variety acts were simply
fillers between the Girl parades. Comedian Will Rogers, who joined
Ziegfeld's revue in 1916, lampooned the show's dynamic: "All these beautiful girls I am the contrast [*sic*]. Somebody has to do something while
[the] girls change clothes even if they dont [*sic*] have much to change." [6]

As the American Girl rhetoric developed around Ziegfeld's *Follies*, the
revue structure suggested an ideology as well as a style. Jewish, ethnic,
and African American comedy, including blackface, in effect functioned
as the "contrast" to the Glorified American Girl. Black comedian Bert
Williams reportedly had a clause in his contract stipulating that he would
never appear on the Ziegfeld stage at the same time as the famous Girls.
For Jewish comedians such as Brice and Eddie Cantor, the difference
from the Glorified Girl was less threatening but made explicit offstage,

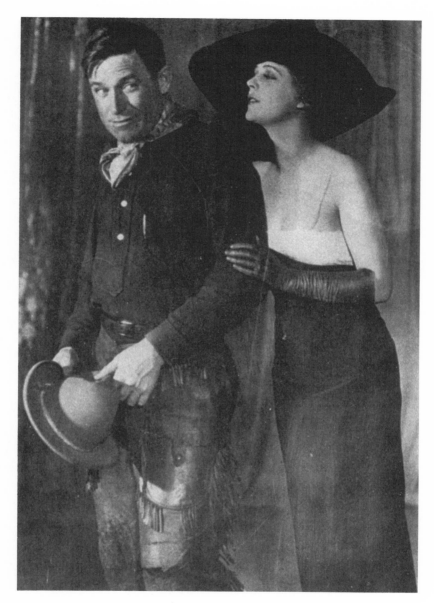

Will Rogers and Follies Girl, circa 1915. "All these beautiful girls I am the contrast [*sic*]. Somebody has to do something while [the] girls change clothes even if they dont [*sic*] have much to change."

in Ziegfeld interviews explaining that his Follies Girls were "native" Americans whose grandparents and great-grandparents had been born in this country. The point of this outrageous fabrication was that Glorified American Girls were not supposed to be recent immigrants from southern and eastern Europe, hence not ethnic, dark-skinned, or Jewish. As camp comedy would do in later years, the boisterous comedy of Fanny Brice mocked these constraints, but Brice's skits also enacted the dynamic described by Will Rogers: "All these beautiful girls I am the contrast."

This ethnic and racial proscription suggests one inflection of the Ziegfeld Girl's bourgeois respectability and, more generally, an example of how female sexuality circulates as a knowledge, discipline, and limit. This knowledge and discipline operates within specific economies. As Hugh Hefner would do much later in the publication world, Ziegfeld produced glossy sexual images as upscale commodities for a middle-class market. Foreshadowings of Hugh Hefner can be glimpsed in certain production numbers — "A Girl for Each Month of the Year," for example, from the 1915 *Follies* — and also in numerous enactments of harems and slave girls: "The Palace of Beauty" from the 1912 edition and "The Treasures of the East" from 1926. These productions of women as art objects or treasured items enabled the occasional topless costume or glimpse of female nudity, justified as an aesthetic touch. Usually, nudity was suggested rather than displayed in the Ziegfeld numbers, and the effect of sheer spectacle always superseded the sheerness of the chiffons.

In fact, the conservative management of the Ziegfeld Girl's sexuality, often noted by her contemporary reviewers, is a clue to her importance in cultural history. The 1912 version featured "a maximum of comely young female shapes with minimum of burdens in way of clothing," one reviewer reported. "But I claim that even the most Puritan man . . . would admit that the sight of all that bare flesh left him cold."[7] The chill was still felt a decade later by Edmund Wilson, who in 1923 described the popularity of the Ziegfeld Girl as "the peculiar frigidity and purity, the frank high-school-girlishness which Americans like." He compared the famous Ziegfeld Walk to military drills: "a row of well-grown girls descends a high flight of stairs in a deliberate and rigid goose-step."[8] As Wilson's point about American Puritanism suggests, the sexuality of

Ziegfeld Girls was regimented and controlled, vacuumed of sweat and passion.

Admirers of the Ziegfeld Walk would dismiss the suggestion it was a "goose-step," but the Walk was certainly a discipline, one of many foregrounded by Ziegfeld in his organization and representations of the Girls. Numerous anecdotes confirm that Ziegfeld was concerned about their offstage behavior, sending them messages about unsuitable dress or behavior on the street and rewarding them for not getting summer suntans. The suntan prohibition—at a time when summer tanning had just become trendy—is a clue to the particularity of the Ziegfeld Girl's body, its meanings and disciplines, its origins, color, and identity. In developing chorus girls who were "real ladies"—that is, respectable white women in public—the Ziegfeld enterprise would eventually define in its advertisements a "distinctly American" girl.

Because this book focuses on the embodiment of a "distinctly American" girl, it is aligned with recent feminist history that aims not to discover and retell stories of lives and events but rather to discover how categories of female sexuality and gender are organized and inscribed in popular images and narratives.[9] My interest includes previous theater history of the Ziegfeld Girl, for example, which often duplicates the awed reception of the original performances. In a 1976 theater history, Robert C. Toll reports that, given an extraordinary lineup of stars such as Fanny Brice, Bert Williams, and Eddie Cantor in the *Follies* of 1917, the "leading attractions were the beautiful, alluring Ziegfeld Girls, the breath-taking, sensational production numbers, and Ann Pennington's dimpled knees."[10] Toll's account continues the assumption that "the beautiful, alluring Ziegfeld Girls" are per se a recognizable and inevitable category rather than an identification created by a certain structure, one that showcases and names "beautiful, alluring Ziegfeld Girls" in contrast to ethnicity, racial difference, and comedy.

Toll is not unaware of the racial implications of Ziegfeld's famous showgirls. "He [Ziegfeld] never said it, but they had to be Caucasians," Toll points out. "Of the some three thousand women he chose to be Ziegfeld Girls, there were no orientals and no Negroes."[11] My own point here is that the racial impact of the *Follies* is not simply the exclusion of color but also the production of whiteness and, specifically, its produc-

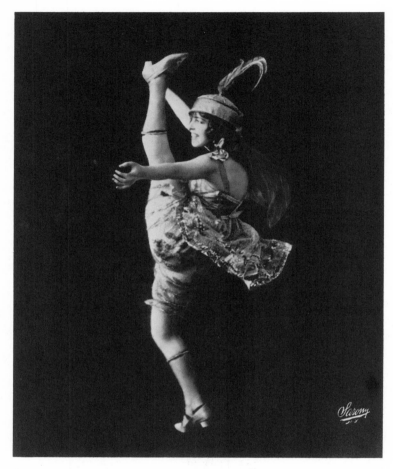

Ann Pennington, dancing star of the *Ziegfeld Follies*, circa 1915. (Billy Rose Theatre Collection, New York Public Library for the Performing Arts)

tion as glamour—the "alluring" women, the "breath-taking" spectacles, the glimpse of Ann Pennington's knees.

Coexisting with the all-black musicals and revues early in the century, and later with the uptown Harlem nightclub entertainers, the posh Ziegfeld Girl performed race as class and as sexuality. Racial whiteness was fetishized through allusions to the light-skinned chorus girls of black Broadway, especially through the marginally scandalous café au lait makeup of certain Ziegfeld Girl performances. In the first *Follies* of 1907, a Follies Girl in café au lait—that is, light-skin or mulatto-effect blackface—sang "Miss Ginger of Jamaica," flaunting herself in the lyrics as an "importation" known for "doing things up brown." Café au lait makeup became a standard sexual mask for the more daring Ziegfeld Girls' performances, a way to appropriate but also to distance a racially structured, forbidden sexuality. Moreover, because the specialty and comedy acts operated as clear contrasts, the Ziegfeld Girl display in the *Follies* show was an enclave of whiteness within a far more racially and ethnically mixed montage of images and stereotypes. The Ziegfeld Girl as a "guarantee" of high quality worked to ensure absolute racial division and definition as well.

The Glorified American Girl was part of a larger conflation of race and nation found in a number of popular discourses of the time. The Ziegfeld era was the age of eugenics, the pseudoscience that posited a Nordic "American race." The Ziegfeld rhetoric of beauty "types" is borrowed from the eugenicist concern with physical "types" and the demarcations of race. Within the eugenicists' arguments, terms of race and ethnicity often blurred to reinforce binary categories of American whiteness and (non-American) nonwhiteness. Even after immigration was stemmed by legislation, postwar racial tensions increased, so that the stakes rose on representations of "the public body" as a white one, giving the whiteness of the Ziegfeld Girl an additional impetus in the 1920s.

The development of the Ziegfeld Girl in the first three decades of this century exemplifies how concepts such as "sexiness" and "glamour" are constituted by these specific class and racial concerns. As historian Peter Bailey has pointed out more recently, glamour is a fairly modern concept involving public visibility of a desirable object, its management or control, and its resulting value as class marker or commodity. The mechanisms of glamour are thus distancing devices that prevent immediate access: the shop window, the cinema screen, the fashion magazine. Bailey emphasizes glamour's dependence on both visibility and inaccessibility, producing the tension of desire.[12] In the United States in the first part of the century, the Broadway revue scene was a prominent site among many cultural practices in which glamour—as certain bodies and certain fashionable products—was being developed. The revues were "the standard to which the American woman looked: they were the most current aesthetic; they were the epitome of style," as the theater historian John Hirsch describes them.[13] Cinema would very quickly rival theater in this development, but the public relations business flaunting theatrical stars and styles was already thriving in the 1890s, when Ziegfeld entered the Broadway revue world and the business of female spectacle.

The word "heterosexuality," as we define it today, is also modern, its contemporary meanings emerging in the latter part of the 1920s, when the word "sexy" also first came into the vocabulary. When a sexuality is packaged as glamour and produced as a commodity, its definitions narrow into class and racial distinctions. The Glorified American Girl is precisely such a distinction and narrowing, a movement toward regulation and standardization of a requisitely white mannequin-showgirl. A specified body, designated as white and heterosexual, was conflated with other desires; the body-we-should-want (as male desire, as female ideal) enacts the other things "we" should want: the society wedding, Anglo blondness, tourism, the Panama Canal.

The Man Who Invented Women: Ziegfeld and the Follies

"The Man Who Invented Women" was the headline of a review of Charles Higham's 1972 biography Ziegfeld. Florenz Ziegfeld Jr. (1868–1932) was not only the producer of twenty-two acclaimed Broadway Follies revues but also nearly as many nightclub Frolic shows and over forty other musicals. To summarize this varied theatrical career as "the invention of women" levels history to hype, but in a fittingly Ziegfeldian way. Its panache borrows from Ziegfeld's history of overstatement and shameless self-promotion, echoing a 1915 news release in which the Ziegfeld persona makes a claim: "I invented the showgirl, and therefore like any other inventor, am qualified to discuss and analyze the child of my brain."[14]

The Ziegfeld name was indeed a trademark, but the showgirl was no Ziegfeld invention. The publicity image of Ziegfeld as Zeus-like captain of industry, emitting showgirls from his forehead, typified the hype surrounding Ziegfeld himself, his Follies extravaganzas, and his high-profile Follies Girl. The 1915 "I invented the showgirl" news release emerged from the keen competition among shows and eponymous showgirls — the Weber and Fields Girl, the Casino Girl, the Shubert Girl, the Dillingham Girl — vying for attention in the thriving revue world of early-twentieth-century Broadway. The 1972 headline, however, acknowledges that Ziegfeld's claim of authority, though overblown in its rhetoric, retained some resonance nearly sixty years later and even expanded its scope, from showgirls to womankind.

The history of the Ziegfeld Girl is inextricable from this history of Ziegfeldian hype and the development of the body as a marketable commodity. Very early in his theatrical ventures, young Ziegfeld supposedly lured an audience to see the Brazilian Invisible Fish — a bowl of water accompanied by a great deal of singsong acclaim. Whether or not this anecdote is true, it became part of the Ziegfeld lore about his wily genius and intuition for drawing a crowd. The point of Woollcott's comment about Ziegfeld's "universal guarantee," quoted above, was that salesmanship of the *Follies* worked on the same principle as the Brazilian Invisible Fish.[15]

During the heyday of the Ziegfeld theatrical enterprise, in recognition of the producer's flair for image and advertisement, his publicists openly flaunted him as "the P. T. Barnum of the theater."[16] Like Barnum, Ziegfeld was always an intriguing background presence during the main event, so the hype or humbug was part of the entertainment package. Hype plays to the combined fascination and suspicion of the consumer and thus always involves fetishization and substitution of the real for the fantasy: "I know better, but. . . ." During the Ziegfeld era, journalists picked up and replayed the Ziegfeld office's own jingoes with a wink and smile, and the posthumous homages to the famous producer and his Girls have tended to restate the same hyperboles. Introducing her 1956 book on the *Follies*, Marjorie Farnsworth typifies the breathless, willing suspension of disbelief: "Women could not possibly be as desirable, beautiful and breath-taking as that," she writes, "yet they were, under the Ziegfeld master touch of illusion."[17]

As Farnsworth's words suggest, marketing, rather than invention, more accurately describes Ziegfeld's genius. His first biographers Eddie Cantor and David Freedman summarized the producer's formula for show business as "one-third glamour, one-third merit, and one-third

advertising."[18] Yet the three elements are hardly separable in the production of the Ziegfeld Girl. Ziegfeld borrowed from previous traditions—the theatrical revue structure, the Americanized operetta girl,
the relatively new celebrity and public relations business—to package
and promote images of women as pricey, nearly unobtainable items—
as glamour. Their value or merit, far from being innate, resided both in
the packaging and in previously established hierarchies of value. "The
man who invented women" was a choreographer of racial, sexual, class,
and consumerist desires that were already present in American culture.
The enduring feature-journalist language of invention, glory, and fairy
tales masks a far more complicated process of how, which, and whose
images and desires are mass-produced and mainstreamed.

The publicity linkage of Ziegfeld to P. T. Barnum was in one sense
literal; Ziegfeld's show business career began in the circus atmosphere
of Buffalo Bill Cody's *Wild West Show,* to which he briefly attached himself as a shooter when he was seventeen. Eschewing his family's world
of classical music, specifically the Chicago Musical College over which
his father presided from 1876 until 1916, Florenz Ziegfeld Jr. was always
more interested in earthier popular entertainment.

Young Ziegfeld's first successful stage sensation was the Great Sandow,
a strongman whom he exhibited in conjunction with the 1893 Chicago
World's Fair. His winning gimmick for Sandow was to open the backstage to allow members of the audience, including the "ladies," to touch
the powerful arm muscles of his star. The Sandow touch-the-flesh ruse
suggests Ziegfeld's strong instinct about the human body as an "attraction" and the increasingly fluid boundaries of respectability in the
middlebrow theater world. The pitch made specifically to the opposite
sex offered a brush of intimacy in a suggestive backstage setting, but
under the auspices of a family amusement show. Female contact with
a stranger's amazing masculine body, a potentially vulgar or dangerous situation, was organized like a tour, safe and public, regulated and
covered by an admission ticket. The Sandow promotion was a touchstone of Ziegfeld's inventiveness at the juncture of the respectable, bourgeois audience and the racy appeal of the flesh—the exact juncture at
which the Ziegfeld Girl as type and ideal would emerge.

The larger juncture here is actually the turn-of-the-century shift

toward new representations and knowledges of the body and its sexualities. During the 1890s, female sexuality in particular was made visible
and commodified in a number of venues, through high-profile, physically sumptuous actresses such as Lillian Russell; through the new female choruses who swayed in the background of musical theater shows;
and through the ubiquitous vaudeville and burlesque appearances of
"women in tights" doing comedy, musical, and acrobatic performances.
Ziegfeld's irrepressible entrepreneurism and his talents for promotion
were well matched with this growing market of female spectacle. He
briefly took Sandow on a road tour after the fair, but in 1896, his attraction to high-style living and company brought him to the social scene of
Broadway's financiers. There Ziegfeld connected with producer Charles
Evans and talked his way into a tour of Europe to find a new musical
actress for a Broadway show. Thus began Ziegfeld's trademark identity
as discoverer and eventually "inventor" of female beauty and stardom.

In 1896, Broadway musical comedy was a robust scene of high-class
consumption and flashy sensationalism. Lively, sometimes risqué theater productions were supported by the sophisticated carriage trade,
the moneyed crowd popularizing the newly developed restaurants and
nightlife of the New York theater district: Rector's, Delmonico's, Sherry's
— the lobster palaces of the Gilded Age. The major components of later
Ziegfeldian theater were already assembled in this milieu. A thoroughly
American popular theater had come into its own, consisting of fast-
paced, often ethnic comedy, vernacular song-and-dance numbers, and
show-stopping visual spectacles (parades, pageantry, or special effects),
the latter of which would develop into the big production numbers of
Broadway and, later, of film musicals.[19] Some of the major figures and
sites of the future Broadway musical-comedy scene had been established
as well. The Shubert brothers produced their first successful slapstick
comedy in 1894, and the first Weber and Fields Music Hall opened in
1896, adding German Jewish comedy to the rowdy Irish comedy previously popularized by Harrigan and Hart musicals.

Broadway was also enjoying two recent imports from France that
additionally enabled the Ziegfeld Girl's evolution: the naughty French
farces, renowned for their suggestive plotlines, and the revue form, the
upscale variety show modeled after the Parisian Moulin Rouge and

Folies Bergère. The farce often featured exotic female stars such as Yvette Guilbert, brought from France by William Hammerstein in 1893, so that scandalous French sensuality (known in America from the "disreputable" novels of Balzac and Zola) was embodied in bewitching actresses for a mainstream audience. The theatrical revue, most notably the *Passing Show,* which opened at the Casino Theater in 1894, also made female sexuality accessible and visible with its inevitable lines of scintillating chorus girls, the theatrical accoutrement that Broadway came to idolize in the next few decades.

The revue form and the developing American musical comedy launched the chorus girl into public prominence in the 1890s. As an emblem of a newly visible female sexuality, this colorful figure remained at the forefront of popular culture well into the 1930s not only as an attractive ingredient of musical theater but also as an established character in popular fiction, plays, and cinema. In her varied manifestations — the diva, the soubrette, and later the clothes model/showgirl — the chorus girl played to a vast cultural imagination and to that imagination's confusion and illusions about female sexuality and about women as workers in a mixed-sex world.

The chorus girl's European antecedents — the operetta girl and the ballet girl, both of whom were more important as visual effects than as musical talent — gave her a slight measure of respectability. She needed no more than an average singing voice and the ability to wear fluffy costumes and a bright smile, but in the 1890s she played in major New York theaters, such as the Knickerbocker, the Casino, the Empire, and therefore was a pricier item than her sisters of the burlesque hall or road-touring vaudeville acts. Journalists of the era began to play up stories of the chorus girl as a titillating version of the era's New Woman — bold, independent, and modern in her attitudes toward men and fun. Although the chorus girl retained the murkier, promiscuous connotations traditionally associated with "theater women," she was also situated within the tantalizing class entitlements of legitimate theater, with its eminently respectable stars such as Lillian Russell, who had "risen from the chorus," as theater lore and magazines such as the *Cosmopolitan* and the *Green Book* frequently emphasized.

This liminal status of the chorus girl in relation to bourgeois respectability was the key to Ziegfeld's articulation and promotion of his Follies Girl. In fact, the immediate predecessor of Ziegfeld's Glorified American Girl was the imported soubrette, the music hall performer whose French origins accorded her some class status. As the envoy of Charles Evans, Ziegfeld ran across musical comedian Anna Held, billed as a Parisian sensation, playing at the Empire Theater in London. Ziegfeld persuaded her to break her contract as a mere *"café-concert"* singer in order to appear in the United States as an *"artiste lyrique."* [20] Held would become famous for such songs as "Won't You Come and Play Wiz Me," but as a Ziegfeld star she played the legitimate theater rather than music halls, demonstrating Ziegfeld's talent for repackaging borderline-risqué material for an upscale venue.

Ziegfeld's 1896 American debut of Anna Held also demonstrated his intuition of hype as the cutting-edge medium of the coming century. Through his orchestration that year, the New York arrival of this European singer was overblown into a months-long news event covered by the major city newspapers as "the comet of the century's end." Her stardom continued for over two decades. Publicized nationwide as the saucy European alternative to the popular American "types" of the day—the Gibson Girl, the statuesque Lillian Russell—the diminutive Held made a reputation for rolling her "misbehaving eyes," shrugging her shoulders, and singing in French—"the naughty language," her daughter Liane Carrera explained years later. In one of her memoirs about her mother, she tells of a man who took his wife to an Anna Held performance on their wedding night. "In such small theaters," she writes suggestively of Held's performances, "one was practically able to touch her." The wedding-night intimacy with Held, says Carrera, was intended to be the bride's lesson on "the facts of life." [21]

Anna Held's daughter, never a fan of Ziegfeld, claims in this same manuscript that Ziegfeld was a carnival-barker at heart. "Without Anna Held it is doubtful that Ziegfeld ever would have thought of glorifying the American Girl," Carrera writes. " 'Little Egypt' the cooch dancer was more in his line." [22] To be fair, there is actually more of a continuum than a clean break between Ziegfeld's touch-the-flesh promotion with Sandow and his promotion of the naughty Anna Held. Both served as a litmus test of how the body and "the facts of life" would be known, seen, and understood at the beginning of a new century. Ziegfeld's ambition and vision, however — particularly his affinity to spectacle — was larger than Held's stardom. Anna Held was reportedly influential in pushing Ziegfeld toward the revue structure of the Parisian *Folies,* but it was perhaps inevitable that he would have been drawn toward this format, especially its grandiose American version.

The revue in the United States had taken a turn toward the spectacular with the 1905 opening of the New York Hippodrome, an immense structure containing restaurants, cafés, and the world's largest stage and theater. Its revues far surpassed the Casino shows in sheer magnitude, interspersing vaudeville-type music and comedy acts with colossal numbers featuring fireworks, panoramas, live elephants, and legions of chorus girls. Ziegfeld used a similar, loosely organized series of music and comedy acts, held together by a gimmicky theme (Captain John Smith and Pocahontas visit New York City) for his first *Follies* show in 1907, which opened at the Jardin de Paris, on the roof of the New York Theater. As the location name suggests, the *Follies* played down the more circuslike aspects of the Hippodrome and drew more on the revue's Parisian precedent. The show's name originated in the satirical skits that, like the New York newspaper column similarly named, drew on the "follies of the day," from Teddy Roosevelt's exploits to Prohibition, which were lampooned or magnified into cartoons or superdramatic enactments. The humor was broad and benign; its targets — personages such as Diamond Jim Brady and Roosevelt himself — eventually appeared in the audience to enjoy the fun. Ziegfeld's revue was immediately a successful annual Manhattan event and soon a nationally known extravaganza: a variety show nearly four hours long that included headliner comedians, singers, dancers, dazzling production numbers, and, of course, the highly publicized Follies Girls.

The *Ziegfeld Follies* shows were staged nearly every year from 1907 to 1931. The stars, comics, and costumes of the *Follies* changed for each annual show, but the structure and the publicity style remained consistent for nearly twenty-two years. Most years, the revue played in New York for the summer and then went on the road, earning rave notices from Pittsburgh to San Francisco. The Ziegfeld publicity machines made certain the show itself and the celebrated Follies Girl became a mainstay of journalism about show business and celebrity. By 1920, Ziegfeld's *Follies* advertised itself as "a National Institution," and in fact, it had by then taken on name recognition far beyond New York City and other urban centers as a symbol for first-class entertainment and female spectacle.

The distinguishing marks of the annual Ziegfeld revues were the lavish production values, Ziegfeld's recruitment of first-rate performers, and the high "quality" of the trademark Girl in the choruses and on the staircase tiers. The Ziegfeld revue also became legendary for characteristics dear to American hype: huge budgets and outrageous one-upmanship. Each year, audiences for the *Follies* looked forward to a concoction that would exceed the previous year's in scope, spectacle, and talent. Ziegfeld's demand for premium materials, stagings, and costumes resulted in over-the-top expenditures, so the show itself did not always make high profits. Nevertheless, the extravagance contributed to the Ziegfeld lore of impeccable taste, the quality that imparted class value to the show and to the Girls.

From its earliest days, the *Follies* banked its reputation on the Girls. In its second year, advertisements for the *Follies* primarily touted a chorus-spectacle show: "Remarkable Cast of 100, with 50 Anna Held Girls, Also the Nell Brinkley Girls, Incomparable Beauty Chorus, the Dancing Dolls." Ziegfeld's 1909 revue was described in the *New York World* as "little less than musical comedy and a little more than vaudeville—a hodge-podge as uncertain as the weather." The reviewer added, however, that "the flock of girls who represented nothing but themselves were [*sic*] the best part of the show." [23]

By 1910, Ziegfeld was referring to the *Follies* as his annual "girl show," and the era's journalists collaborated in this acclaim. The *New York Star* described the 1909 *Follies* as "girls, girls and then more girls, with comedians galore . . . a wealth of fun and music and girls piled mountain-high each on each." Five years later, a *New York Times* review used virtually the same language, admitting that the 1914 *Follies* show was "dangerously close to the border line of stupidity, but there are girls and girls and girls and plenty of real comedians and many more real dancers," so that "all is forgiven." [24] The *New York American*, the newspaper of Ziegfeld's friend Randolph Hearst, faithfully reviewed the *Follies* each year as girl shows, illustrating the annual offering with two-column photos of Zieg-

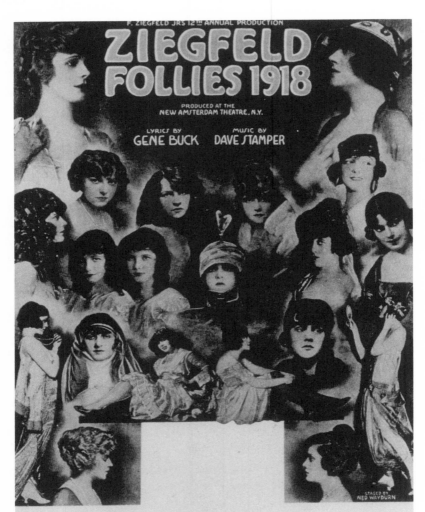

Advertisement for the *Ziegfeld Follies* of 1918.

feld beauties. Chorus-stricken *New York World* journalist Roy J. McCardell ensured that adequate coverage was given to the annual "crop" of Girls with weekly stories, teasing readers as the revue season began and reminding them, during the long winters, that chorus girls were blooming somewhere outside New York and would be ripe for picking soon.

Anna Held never appeared in the *Follies*, for by 1907 Ziegfeld was interested in a different type, a taller woman who could better display grandiose costumes. In the early years of the Ziegfeld revues, the chorus line was called the Anna Held Girls to conjure some of the French star's exotic allure. But Ziegfeld's delectable music hall soubrette quickly evolved into the long-legged American beauty, glossy and untouchable. This is the version of the chorus girl who would become a highlight of the annual *Follies* show, famous for her signature entrance on a staircase and her runway exhibition of the Ziegfeld Walk, a combination of pageantry strut and haute couture modeling. The Ziegfeld office preferred to call her "the showgirl" rather than the chorus girl. Whereas chorus girls danced and kicked, showgirls glided and posed. Technically, both were Ziegfeld Girls, but the latter—specifically associated with high-class fashion—would be the linchpin of the Ziegfeld legend and enterprise.

After 1915, with the hiring of Viennese stage designer Joseph Urban and international fashion designer Lucile Duff Gordon, the *Follies'* focus shifted even further toward spectacular visual effects featuring the Girls. Under the direction of Duff Gordon, the Ziegfeld Girl was specifically linked to haute couture fashion, with some of Duff Gordon's models hired as *Follies* showgirls. In the earlier *Follies* programs, the chorus girls sometimes interacted with the audience by tossing balloons and candies. But the more remote, elegant showgirl of the later *Follies,* modeling upscale fashions within sumptuous settings, would become Ziegfeld's brand-name woman performer. The consensus of revue theater historians is that she "set a new standard not only for chorus lines of other revues but for parading mannequins everywhere." [25]

The showgirl pageants included processions and musical performances, climaxing with a stunning tableau. Within Urban's elaborate stagings, teams of women's bodies served as architectural background, historical backdrop, or aesthetic designs, while other teams promenaded or danced in the foreground. The themes of these spectacles provide an index of cultural fantasies and preoccupations in the first three decades of the century: the Gibson Girl from contemporary images, Arabian harems from the era's Orientalist inclinations, jaunty showgirl versions of the New Woman as aviator or acrobat. Often the theme was a whimsical or artistic one — "Melody, Fantasy, and the *Follies* of Years Gone By" or imitations of classic paintings that required quantities of elaborately costumed bodies, with the occasional, tasteful glimpse of bare breast. Mininarratives often structured these pageants enacting Cleopatra's romance or springtime in Paris, but their point was visual: ornamental women and settings, breathtaking costumes, opulent special effects.

No matter how talented the annual lineup of comedy and musical stars proved to be, the reputation of the Ziegfeld revue as a girl show was virtually clinched by the "Glorified American Girl" motto of the 1920s. Furthering this emphasis, legends and rumors accumulated about Ziegfeld's own bias toward portions of the show featuring the Girls. Will Rogers may have been joking about biding time for the showgirls, but theatrical histories document Ziegfeld's concern at least on some occasions that comedy skits should be timed around "the girls'" costume changes.[26] One of the issues in Ziegfeld biographies and journalists' reports is whether he appreciated the talent of notables such as Rogers, Eddie Cantor, W. C. Fields, and other players who went on (generally to Hollywood) as stars. "When Mr. Ziegfeld laughs even once, it's news," the *New York Times* reported toward the end of his career. "If he does it again, it's a contract." The most popularly repeated anecdotes suggest he never stopped equating the *Follies* with the Girls. After Ziegfeld's death, one of his writers claimed it was typical of the producer to interrupt comedy skit rehearsals in order to get to the parade of showgirls. "That's enough," Ziegfeld would say. "Bring on the girls." [27]

Testifying to this same inclination of Ziegfeld during the preparations for *Show Boat*, Oscar Hammerstein II vowed never to do another show with him because the great producer was so preoccupied with visual effects, particularly the visual effects of the chorus girls. Trying to consult with Ziegfeld about some major structural changes during a rehearsal, Hammerstein found him with "a faraway look" in his eyes, calling to a girl onstage, "I like the way you had your hair done yesterday." Critic Gilbert Seldes in 1931 similarly reported that Ziegfeld was willing to hold up rehearsals while he fussed with a chorus girl's ribbon or hat. According to Seldes, at the end of his career Ziegfeld was still discounting the twenty-some years of talented comedy and musical routines in the *Follies*. "To him they are still girl shows."[28]

The ubiquity of the anecdotes may simply confirm the public's own preoccupations. After relating one such cut-the-comedy story in his newspaper column, Ed Sullivan claims Ziegfeld telephoned him to protest and remind him how many comedy stars the *Follies* had launched. "There's something more to my shows than beautiful girls, despite what they say," Ziegfeld reportedly told him.[29] Yet "what they say"—the folkloric reputation of the *Follies* as the production of Girls—is very much part of the *Follies'* lived history, parallel to the theatrical history of the Ziegfeld's comic/music stars and their multiple success stories. If anything, "what they say" suggests how powerfully this version of female sexuality, packaged as brand-name showgirl, was inscribed in the public imagination.

Hype to Homage

The Ziegfeld publicity office regularly played up the power and mystery of Ziegfeld's judgments about female beauty. "He is a man whom many visit, but whom few see," a 1923 news release reported. "Behind a magnificent desk in a gorgeously furnished room on the ninth floor of the New Amsterdam Theater Building he sits and passes judgment." In an essay written that same year, theater critic George Jean Nathan declared Ziegfeld an artist on the same plane as Dostoevsky and Stanislavsky and praised Ziegfeld's "hocus-pocus" in materializing a sophisticated but innocent chorus girl: "Little Bright Eyes from the spiritual world, dressed in thin black stockings and pink garters." Countless journalists and interviewers asked, "How does he do it?" "Where does he get his girls?" "How can he pick them?" In response, the Ziegfeld office released countless news releases—"How I Judge Beauty," "How to Be a Ziegfeld Girl"—each mystifying the process in a rhetoric of "glorification" and "pulchritude." J. P. McEvoy, one of his writers, eulogized his boss in 1932 with the familiar litany of questions and puzzlement: "I have watched him pick girls for the *Follies* and I can't tell you how he picked them. What did he look for? I don't know. . . . Ziegfeld's eye for detail was miraculous."[30]

In short, the rhetoric positioned Ziegfeld and his Girls in artistic and even mythic terms, with significance beyond mere entertainment. The "Glorifying the American Girl" motto reinforced the power and artistic vision of the Glorifier. The wording appeared frequently in reviews and headlines: "Follies Glorify Girlish Beauty," "Miss Lange has been on Broadway only nine months and already is glorified." Apparently the rhetoric was taken seriously within the Ziegfeld office. Seldes reported that " 'glorified' is in the Ziegfeld office the common and preferred synonym for 'in the chorus.' You hear 'she was glorified in 1921,' or 'she hasn't been glorified since 1924,' and there is neither self-consciousness nor irony in the expression."[31]

The motto inscribed on every *Follies* theater program beginning in 1922, "A National Institution—Glorifying the American Girl," was supplemented on the 1927 program with the maxim, "He who glorifies beauty glorifies truth." Theater reviewer J. Brooks Atkinson commented that the "bold" proclamation about "truth" on the 1927 program was given "real substance" by the showgirls and show.[37] That is, the myth-making about the producer and his project may have originated with Ziegfeld's publicity office, but it was enthusiastically complemented by reviewers such as Atkinson and Nathan—writers for upscale national journals—as well as local journalists for city newspapers and tabloids.

As late as 1930, when the *Follies* show was in serious financial trouble, it was still being described by a Los Angeles reviewer as a revered national institution symbolized by the eponymous showgirl: "Ziegfeld Girls, often well educated, nearly always well mannered, have supplied the last word in beauty and costume for newspaper and magazine illustrations for years. The Ziegfeld *Follies,* like apple pie, ham and eggs . . . is a distinctly American institution. It is the only permanent theater idea in the United States."[33]

In fact, neither the *Follies* idea nor the Ziegfeld showgirl became permanent on Broadway. Even the most fawning biographers of Ziegfeld admit that the *Follies'* theatrical formula had reached its limits by the

1930s. The revue structure itself was being replaced in popularity by the integrated narrative musical, a form newly replicated by sound technology in motion pictures. Ziegfeld's high-budget revues not only outpriced themselves but faced the competition of talking motion pictures, which could reproduce the chorus girl for wider audiences and far lower ticket prices by the late 1920s. Ever the cutting-edge entrepreneur, Ziegfeld in his last years was himself involved in the production of integrated musicals such as *Sally* and *Show Boat* and in motion pictures, although he never got himself out of debt or recovered from the stock market crash of 1929. Ziegfeld produced his last *Follies* in 1931 and died in 1932. Over the next few years, his widow, Billie Burke, coproduced some *Follies* shows with the Shuberts, and through the 1950s, *Follies*-type revues sporadically ran on Broadway, although these shows never attained the status and success of the originals.

Almost immediately after Ziegfeld's death, however, the legends of his grand revue and guaranteed Girl were again taken up and aggrandized in popular media, including Hollywood musicals, the very form that helped to bury the Ziegfeld-style theatrical tradition. The "permanent theater idea" of Ziegfeld is thus the legend of an extravagant producer/artist and a glamorous showgirl/art object — Glorifier and Glorified. It is not simply that the hype has outlasted the enterprise but also that the hype — as promotion and gimmick — has been converted into a more earnest and nostalgic rhetoric about women, glamour, and American images.

The Ziegfeld glorified/glorifier mythology was given full-scale treatment and authority in the affectionate 1934 biography *Ziegfeld, the Great Glorifier,* by Eddie Cantor and David Freedman. Because Cantor was a Ziegfeld star and friend, this first biography is unsurprisingly eulogistic and deferential, praising Ziegfeld as the "inventor" of "American Beauty . . . the Knight Errant of American Womanhood." [34] Its anecdotes about Ziegfeld's personal life, which publicists had dropped into news releases for the previous quarter century, are loosely gathered here as testaments to artistic quirkiness. Ziegfeld's pickiness about his personal clothing, his private railway car, his obsessive micromanagement of the shows, and other eccentricities are offered as proofs of his genius. Cantor and Freedman's picture of Ziegfeld as a benign, somewhat dapper artist and inventor of American beauty was especially influential in the 1936 film *The Great Ziegfeld,* down to the amazing details of the producer's deathbed hallucination of one final grand revue, a scene not to be missed by MGM. Because the film won the Academy Award as Best Picture of 1936, it more generally won a place in film history that further legitimized the Cantor-Freedman version of Ziegfeld as Glorifier and the women stars as products of a superior theatrical mastermind.

The MGM biopic recharged nostalgic journalistic attention to the *Follies,* its producer, and its Girl. The films *Ziegfeld Girl* and *The Ziegfeld Follies* in the 1940s spawned yet another wave of publicity-related feature stories: "The Girls Who Glorified Ziegfeld," "This Was Ziegfeld," "Nostalgia Prevails for Ziegfeld *Follies.*" Journalists such as Adele Rogers St. John still used the glorification metaphor seamlessly at this time: "His name has become part of the English language as has that of no other stage producer . . . above all in the glorification of the American girl which he began." Through the next two decades, the Ziegfeld Girl remained a splendid bank on which magazines such as *Life* could draw human interest stories around photo spreads: "Ziegfeld Girls Recall the Fun of the *Follies*" or "Ziegfeld Girls Hold a Reunion."[35] Supplementing the biographical details of the producer himself, in 1949 Billie Burke published a memoir, *With a Feather on My Nose,* furthering the beloved portrait of Ziegfeld as an extravagant artist and paternal caretaker of his shows and his Girls.

The next major documentation continued this tradition of homage as history. Farnsworth's amply illustrated book *The Ziegfeld Follies* shifted emphasis from Ziegfeld to the shows, providing the first detailed account and chronology of the revues and Ziegfeld's other productions. This is also the first history of the Girls, organized as accolades to the successful ones who headlined programs or who went on to fame in other entertainment venues. As suggested earlier in this introduction, Farnsworth's tone is rhapsodic, naturalizing both producer and Girl as objects of idolization. The Farnsworth book also continued the mystification of the audition and selection process, describing "the magic 'You' in the high-pitched voice of Ziegfeld as he sat in the orchestra's first row center and scanned the hundreds of aspirants." Farnsworth positions the *Follies* show as a heaven of celebrity, with Ziegfeld as its god who "opened the gates to a legendary realm for the most famous girls the world has ever known."[36]

The disembodied voice, the call of selection, has in this way been aggrandized as a sign of power.[37] Ziegfeld would be represented as this voice, the call from the dark, in a number of films and in the 1991 Broadway musical *The Will Rogers Follies*. The disembodiment further empowers the Ziegfeld figure by emphasizing the dynamics of an invisible observer for the showgirl display. For nearly a century, popular culture has apparently been enchanted by Ziegfeld's magical call of selection pinpointing "the most famous girls the world has ever known." The "You" addressed not just a particular successful aspirant but also a more encompassing mass audience ready to nod, to acquiesce in the obvious status of the Ziegfeld Girl as ideal sexual and social body.

In 1957, the fifty-first anniversary edition of *Variety* honored Ziegfeld with an extensive and celebratory history summarizing each of the *Follies* in more detail than had been done either by Cantor and Freedman or by Farnsworth.[38] The author of this history, theater chronicler Robert Baral, followed up with the 1962 book *Revue: A Nostalgic Reprise of the Great Broadway Period*, which situates the Ziegfeld show as the paradigm and paragon of the revue tradition. Often using the grandiose language of the Farnsworth book, it enshrines Ziegfeld not only as "Great Glorifier" but as "ruler de facto of the Beauty Trust" during this era, an echo of Ziegfeld publicity about the trademark Girl and about Ziegfeld himself as captain of industry. The Baral history names the theme song of the revue era as Irving Berlin's "A Pretty Girl Is Like a Melody," originally used in the 1919 *Follies* and immortalized in the 1936 film *The Great Ziegfeld*. The book's final illustration, three photographs of all-girl *Follies* pageant scenes, bears a caption referencing the well-known Ziegfeld anecdote, "Bring on the girls."[39] My point here is that history, nostalgia, legend, and cinema had tightened the loop by 1962, each pointing to the other as evidence, so that the meanings and significance of Ziegfeld as Glorifier seemed obvious and irrefutable.

The centralization of Ziegfeld and the Girls as the meaning of the *Follies* continues in the first serious biography, Charles Higham's *Ziegfeld* (1972). Higham, whose perspective was rooted in Hollywood journalism and pop Freudianism, was far less in awe of the Ziegfeld enterprise than were Cantor and Freedman, Farnsworth, and Baral. His more distanced tone and the current mores of journalism enabled racier details to come forward, including for the first time the less-than-saintly accounts about Ziegfeld's nearly constant affairs with his women stars. According to Higham, the *Follies* spectacles were enactments not just of male fantasy but also of Ziegfeld's "essentially primitive sexual character. The *Follies* were astonishing demonstrations of the mind of a man who sought to release his need for women in displays of adulation for them." [40] Jammed with Freudian speculations and lively anecdotes, this biography delivers the *Follies* history as personal history, with the assumption that "primitive sexual character" — a biological urge — was the trajectory of a thirty-year theatrical enterprise.

Randolph Carter's *Ziegfeld: The Time of His Life* (1974) disdains the psychological interpretations and focuses instead on theater history and iconography. As a primarily visual account of the Ziegfeld years, this book gives as much illustration space to the sets, stage interiors, and theater facades as to the images of the women. For Carter, the Ziegfeld enterprise was about art rather than sex; specifically, it was about the complementary artistries of Ziegfeld and set designer Joseph Urban. Thus his text hurries through the (by then) well-known biographical accounts with the assumption that readers will be more interested in the lavish illustrations, including color prints of Urban's painted sets. What the Carter book shares with Higham's biography, however, is its centralization of Ziegfeld as the vision and genius through which we can understand a theater era or "time of his life." Ziegfeld's "incredible dynamic energy" and "almost superhuman impulsion," Carter admits, can as easily describe "Wagner, Balzac, Florence Nightingale, Adolf Hitler, to mention but a few." [41] For Carter as well as for Higham, a historical era can best be described through the prism of the one dynamic individual whose "superhuman impulsion" creates art, chaos, or both.

In Ziegfeldian bigger-and-better tradition, the recent biographies have each tended to top the last in detail, production values, and glossy design. Whereas Higham's book provided the first frank perspective of the producer's life, Carter's book splendidly illustrated it and was reprinted as an attractive paperback in 1988. The most recent Ziegfeld tome exceeds both books in biographical detail and lush photographic evidence. This is Richard and Paulette Ziegfeld's *The Ziegfeld Touch,* a sumptuous coffee-table volume that includes short biographies of the featured players, 375 illustrations, and 67 full-color plates. Meticulous in its research and presentation of evidence, *The Ziegfeld Touch* is a formidable accumulation of the smallest details of this legendary show business enterprise. Like its predecessors, it presumes and addresses a continued cultural fascination for the producer, the shows, and the Girls. The authors (Richard Ziegfeld is a distant cousin) painstakingly document Ziegfeld's accomplishments, theatrical innovations, and personal life without attempting a psychological or social framework. Its framework instead is entertainment: the book is organized into two "acts" with an "intermission" of thirty-one pages of color-print posters, sheet music covers, and other illustrations.

Hence the "glorifying" language of the original Ziegfeld enterprise is used fairly seamlessly as a way to describe Ziegfeld's work. "Ziegfeld's consummate accomplishment was to glorify women in ways that appealed to both sexes," the authors conclude, correcting the earlier "girlie" appeal described by Baral. The Ziegfelds also admit that "today, Ziegfeld's glorification of women provides ambivalent reactions. In his day, though, the attention he lavished upon women was one step in the process of bringing women into the center of society." [42] Questions of *which* women or *which* center of society are outside the scope of *The Ziegfeld Touch,* which is grounded on a priori assumptions about the Ziegfeld Girl as a self-evident "consummate accomplishment" of the famous showman.

Despite ongoing camp treatments of the Ziegfeld enterprise in the 1990s, *The Ziegfeld Touch* exemplifies how a mainstream reverence persists as well. The 1996 *New York Times* article cited at the beginning of this introduction refers to Ziegfeld's "glorious specimens of American womanhood" with affection rather than irony. Even a more scholarly 1994 retrospect on Ziegfeld's showgirl describes her importance and Americanization without interrogating the terms or premises of this phenomenon. In an article in *American Scholar,* Michael Lasser reiterates Ziegfeld's significance as the man who "shaped the American perception of female beauty" and "showed all of us that no one could be as magnificent as a *Follies* Girl." His conclusion is that American showgirls never again attained this status "without Ziegfeld's adoration and the gift of his transforming imagination."[43] The admiring tone of these passages hearkens back to George Jean Nathan's awe of Ziegfeld's "hocus-pocus" and, earlier than that, to the Ziegfeld publicity office's flaunting of showgirls as children of the genius-inventor's brain.

The Ziegfeld enterprise has remained alive in other popular media as well. As I describe in detail in Chapter 5, Hollywood's own histories and reinscriptions of Ziegfeld are substantial. With modified spectacle but ample melodrama, made-for-TV movies celebrate the Ziegfeld glitz at least once a decade. On Broadway, a play about a reunion of Ziegfeld Girls eventually became Harold Prince's 1971 Follies. In London, a $7 million musical production, Ziegfeld, briefly played in 1988. "Ziegfeld is still a name which sparkles in people's memories, even over here," its writer, Ned Sherrin, explained.[44] The 1989 musical Ziegfeld: A Night at the Follies featured an extravaganza of three hundred costumes and a plotline recycled from decades of Ziegfeld clichés: small-town girls, ambitions for the bright lights, and an affinity for glitzy headdresses. And in its years on Broadway and on tour in the 1990s, The Will Rogers Follies featured Florenz Ziegfeld's voice emanating powerfully from a dark upper tier in the theater, spoken by the recorded voice of Gregory Peck.

For my own purposes, the Ziegfeld described in this book is this haunting voice from the back of the dark theater, the mythological "permanent theater idea." My use of the name "Ziegfeld" for the most part refers not so much to the historical person as to this persona and its hieroglyphic meanings as opulence and spectacle. In Ziegfeld's press releases, this persona has showgirls streaming out of his head, and in the 1936 MGM biopic, they salute him on his deathbed in one last grand revue. Biographies have amply investigated the historical person, but this persona has remained preordained and inalienable, hooked inevitably to its "consummate achievement," the Ziegfeld Girl.

The 1972 book review headline "The Man Who Invented Women" may point to its own silliness with a big wink, but it also acknowledges Ziegfeld in retrospect as the foremost showbiz daddy of his day. In the long run, Ziegfeld's rival Broadway producers — George White, Earl Carroll, the Shuberts, all resoundingly successful in their own right — never generated the legendary discourse that developed and continues to circulate around Ziegfeld and his Girl. While Ziegfeld's hype aimed to sell tickets, this long-term rhetoric persuades us to invest in larger cultural images and identities.

Contexts, Themes, Frameworks

This book focuses on the four major developments in Ziegfeld's theatrical enterprise that defined and circulated the Glorified American Girl: the influence of Anna Held as a template of glamour at the turn of the century; Ziegfeld's repackaging of the chorus girl as bourgeois body in the early *Follies;* the development of the fashion-model Follies Girl after 1915; and the specifically racialized showgirl produced by the later *Follies* in direct response to pressures of immigration and black Broadway. In the last chapter of the book I examine these issues in a number of Hollywood films, the site where the Ziegfeld Girl has probably been most familiarized for contemporary audiences.

As these topics indicate, the voyeuristic dynamic of the Ziegfeld Girl project is not my primary concern here, even though Ziegfeld's own metaphors of invention and glorification strongly suggest male fantasy, specifically, male fantasy of the control of women. The claim of a powerful male producer to have "invented the showgirl" as child of his brain, even if understood as public relations hyperbole, could also be understood as male anxiety and disavowal. Moreover, the excessive costuming and display in the Ziegfeld showgirl performances suggests an almost literal enactment of male voyeuristic fantasy. Parading across the stage in elaborate headdresses and outrageous outfits designed to portray everything from chandeliers to fruits and battleships, the Ziegfeld Girl vividly demonstrates the fetish, the substitute object.

As male fantasy, the Ziegfeld Girl in choreographed parade seems to function as pure "to-be-looked-at-ness," as described in Laura Mulvey's well-known essay on female spectacle in cinema. Mulvey describes the "device of the show-girl" as an example of the visual sexual dynamics of cinema, a justification for the woman to perform directly to the camera as sexual display. Mulvey, in fact, mentions Ziegfeld and choreographer Busby Berkeley, at one time an apprentice to Ziegfeld, as important agents of the showgirl device.[45] Ziegfeld's influence on the Hollywood backstage musical has been widely acknowledged. Rick Altman describes the gender dynamics of the backstage musical in particular as a Ziegfeldesque formula: "man = eyes = camera = desire; woman = body = art = object of desire."[46] Such moments of female spectacle temporarily stop the unfolding of the story, positioning the sexualized woman outside the film's narrative dynamic. The Broadway revues were structured this way as well, the elaborate showgirl numbers bringing to a standstill the faster pace of the comic monologues and skits. To extend this model, we could imagine the theatrical Ziegfeld Girl parading outside more serious ongoing historical and political narratives, as a comforting alternative to threatening female figures of the time: the New Woman, the suffragist, the flapper, the vamp.

Certainly the voyeuristic appeal of this showgirl makes the psychosexual explanation compelling. But the Ziegfeld Girl as male fantasy is too narrow an explanation for the Ziegfeld Girl as glamour, which immediately involves race, class, and, most obviously, female consumers/spectators. Women in the audience were crucial for the success of the *Follies* as an upscale venue and showcase display window. The Ziegfeld Girl's association with high-class clothing in the early *Follies* and her more developed identification as a fashion icon after 1915 were specifically aimed at this portion of the audience.

In addition, the Ziegfeld Girl was not necessarily a static, clear-cut alternative to more threatening figures in women's history during this era. The showgirl as independent working woman represented contentious issues of female public visibility, including newly visible issues of both lesbianism and heterosexual female desire. The Ziegfeld Girl's promotion as the Glorified American Girl connects her to the supposedly progressive New Woman by way of the latter's racial purification concerns.[47] To imagine the revue business as female spectacle and male spectatorship implies a monolithically male investment in the issues of race and nationalism enacted by the Ziegfeld Girl. The danger here is a misinterpretation of racial and national categories as masculinist in their origins, as if white women did not participate in the formations of these identities. My focus, then, on the issues of glamour, commodification, race, and nationalism acknowledges that middle- and upper-class white female audiences had a direct stake in the Ziegfeld Girl's meanings and circulation.

This book begins the Ziegfeld Girl history, in Chapter 1, with Ziegfeld's first female celebrity, Anna Held. At the margins of the Ziegfeld Girl enterprise, Held's career is significant for what it expressed and what it excluded. Her success suggests Ziegfeld's timeliness in producing cutting-edge female images in the early twentieth century, the popular personalities who sold not just theater tickets but also clothing styles and ideas about self and society. Current scholarship, especially in film studies, has explored stardom and celebrity as cultural means of "making sense of the experience of being a person in a particular kind of social production," as Richard Dyer has put it.[48] Held's career also vividly illustrates the racial and ethnic dimensions of this dynamic. Held was born in Warsaw of a French Jewish father and Polish Catholic mother, and she began her show business career in Yiddish theater in London. But Ziegfeld repackaged Held into the fashionable Parisian chanteuse, source of chic advice to American women about French cosmetics and corsetry. Rumors about her Jewish identity and place of birth often haunted her and directed her stylization into a specific exoticized image. Held's meaning as "the facts of life," then, was both a bleaching and a commodification of those facts, illustrating how "glamour" as white and western European in origin worked as racial erasure and definition.

Chapter 2 describes Ziegfeld's entry into the turn-of-the-century "cult of the chorus girl" and the development of his showgirl, beginning with the 1907 *Follies*, as a defined and managed model of female heterosexuality. In this chapter I also address the specifically sexual implications of Ziegfeld Girl management and discipline. First, the pressure to discern "real ladies" from "women of the streets" had become more urgent as the public presence of women increased in the first decades of this century, in the workplace and in social sites such as the department store and the amusement park. The chorus girl exemplified "a line of working women" whose meanings were specifically sexual. Addressing a middle- to upper-class audience, the Ziegfeld publicity and the shows themselves constantly oscillated between the racy and the respectable to tantalize this audience without transgressing images of acceptable female sexuality. Second, the Ziegfeld Girl exemplified female heterosexuality itself as defined and knowable during the first two decades of this century, as lesbianism was slowly being identified as a category, first by sexologists and later in more widely circulated media. Hence the high-profile Ziegfeld Girl body as wholesome ideal, bound for marriage (to a millionaire, according to often repeated media stories), worked as one way to stabilize changing concepts of female sexuality—indeed, fitting them to a "trademark" and a "guarantee."

The *Follies'* move toward haute couture fashion after 1915 is the focus of Chapter 3. The revue itself eventually operated as a showroom or display window, with the trademark Girls modeling designer clothes, accessories, and living styles. The Ziegfeld era encompasses the period documented by historian William R. Leach as the "crucial formative years" of consumer capitalism in the United States, characterized by a "commercial aesthetic" evident in the new materials for advertisement and showcase display: "the visual materials of desire—color, glass, light." Describing the Ziegfeld's Girl's studied respectability, Robert C. Allen precisely locates her within this showroom culture of display, where signs of class and fashion merge with ideals of sexuality, studded with the glittery materials of desire.[49] Show, showgirl, and other commodities were conflated into one highly valued package.

Fashion as a cultural and economic dynamic perhaps illustrates most powerfully how the Ziegfeld Girl as "model" was innately constituted by issues of race. This is not surprising considering the spirited rebirth of the Ku Klux Klan in the second decade of this century. The Ziegfeld publicity discourses were part of the larger nationalization of an Anglicized ideal of beauty, a response to heightened immigration before 1920 and racial tensions in the next decade. The development of a black entertainment business during this era, especially in Manhattan theater, increased the pressure to define "true" glamour—that is, white sexuality—on Broadway. In Chapter 4 I argue that the reverse was true as well: that the glamorous space on Broadway worked as one definition of whiteness, with the generic showgirl as a key element in this definition and the Ziegfeld Girl as its foremost exponent.

My concluding chapter examines the Ziegfeld Girl's legacy in Hollywood cinema, the mode through which most audiences since 1930 have known the Ziegfeld enterprise. Sound cinema—specifically, the backstage musical—usurped the place of theatrical revues such as Ziegfeld's, but cinema also glorified and immortalized Ziegfeld and his Girl, ensuring them both a prominent place in popular cultural history. Ziegfeld's own ventures into film production are covered in this chapter, as are the two major "historical" films, *The Great Ziegfeld* and *Ziegfeld Girl,* that offer Hollywood versions of the Glorifier and the Glorified. The latter two films also illustrate the complexity of the Ziegfeld showgirl's social positioning. Whereas the *Great Ziegfeld* biopic delivers a coherent hero and narrative line, the representation of *the* Ziegfeld Girl in the other film is fragmented into three conflicting characters and stories, suggesting the Glorified Girl's impossible status as ideal and icon. Chapter 5 concludes with a discussion of the Busby Berkeley showgirl, as Hollywood's most logical match of Ziegfeld stylistics and cinematic spectacle. Finally, my epilogue addresses 1990s readings and representations of the Ziegfeld Girl, especially the camp interpretations of her cinematic history.

I am indebted to several strong models of scholarship that have enabled me to address these topics—race and sexual identity, commodification and celebrity—as continuums. By postulating that the Ziegfeld Girl was neither incidentally nor obviously white, I am relying on recent studies of the "inventions" of race and the institutionalization of whiteness. As presented by Theodore W. Allen and others, this scholarship contends that the privileging of one race over another occurs in organized ways (not as "natural" divisions based on appearance and skin color) and becomes effective through particular social establishments. Allen's primary example is English prejudice against the Irish, a case in which skin color fails to explain a racism more explicable through a history of systematic oppression. Recent cultural scholarship, following this line of reasoning, has begun to examine popular texts and entertainment traditions as "racialized," not necessarily racist but structured by racial assumptions. For these studies, white female imagery has been of particular interest because it has symbolized concepts such as nationalism, civilization, morality, and purity, themes that have been significant in implementations of racial thinking.[50]

The assumed whiteness and heterosexuality of the Ziegfeld Girl were not parallel but intersecting issues and concerns. If Ziegfeld Girls were classified as valuable commodities, it was because their value as "American"—that is, as white—was also their heterosexual value. In her 1994 work on the "racial matrix" of culture, Laura Doyle points out how race and sexuality were closely connected in eugenicist concerns for "pure" whiteness in the early part of this century. The role of the reproductive woman — the heterosexual white woman in a legitimate marriage — was a key issue in anxieties about racial purity. Using an anthropological model, Doyle illustrates how "dominant group men create and disseminate images of women that mirror and reinforce the actual circulation of women."[51]

Investigating representation in visual media, Richard Dyer's *White* (1997) similarly emphasizes the junction of race and sexuality. "If race is always about bodies," he reminds us, "it is also always about the reproduction of those bodies through heterosexuality." Dyer's case studies include ubiquitous conventions of photography and film lighting — that is, conventions that have been naturalized or considered "neutral," as if whiteness were a universal and all-inclusive standard. "The idea of whiteness as neutrality already suggests its usefulness for designating a social group that is to be taken for the human ordinary," Dyer points out.[52] As a highly visible ideal or type of body literally "on show," the Ziegfeld Girl's racial and sexual identification was a crucial element of her "guaranteed" quality and value.

Although the function of female imagery is one of the oldest themes in feminist scholarship, more recent work on this topic by Martha Banta and Lois W. Banner influenced my focus and inquiries. The term "Ziegfeld Girl" operated within a national discourse that had produced other brand-name girls from the 1890s to the 1930s: the Gibson Girl, the Christy Girl, the Floradora Girl, the Weber and Fields Girl. As Banta and Banner have persuasively illustrated, these images represented not just varying physical ideals but also contentious ideological questions concerning the changing roles of women, shifts in traditional values, and the defining of "the American" in an era of racial tensions and increased immigration from southern and eastern Europe. In *Imaging American Women*, Banta analyzes the iconic significance of popular female images between 1876 and 1918, especially the importance of cultural "types" as sites of social conflict. Female imagery became the litmus test of "true" Americanism, Banta argues. She includes the Ziegfeld Girl as one of many social signs of American womanhood developed in the wake of a rapidly changing culture in which the idea of a monolithic Americanism was being challenged. At the same time, she points out, industrialization and media technologies were making standardization possible and desirable. My aim here is to amplify one piece of Banta's work by examining in detail how the Ziegfeld enterprise functioned as one such standardization that is still culturally idealized. Likewise, my study develops one of the types or images enumerated by Banner in *American Beauty*, a history of how concepts of female beauty, far from being universal or timeless, are historically and socially derived. Banner is especially enlightening in illustrating how cultural ideals are often not imposed from a higher class but emerge from more popular roots, such as female athletes and chorus girls.[53]

Examining a very different kind of female spectacle, Robert C. Allen's landmark study of American burlesque scrupulously traces what he calls the "intelligibility" of the burlesque tradition and performance. Although the connotations of this theater tradition may lean toward the lurid or even the pornographic, Allen demonstrates that its meanings, interpretations, and effects were never so monolithic. Drawing on the work of Mikhail Bakhtin, Michel Foucault, and Victor Turner, Allen explores the paradoxes of this theatrical tradition without attempting to claim it as "ultimately" either transgressive or exploitative in relation to female sexuality. No single reading of burlesque accounts for its contradictions and various positionings within culture, he argues. Yet this theatrical practice, as rendered by Allen, tells us a great deal about struggles and crises of gender, class, and race relations in the last part of the nineteenth century, providing a rich contribution to the history of women and gender in America. Allen locates the Ziegfeld Girl as a marker ending burlesque's rowdy history, citing her icy respectability and onstage silence as a nonthreatening version of female spectacle.[54] Like Allen, I aim to read a past performance tradition as a text, a case study that examines one local practice and its accompanying discourses.

To ask the question of how burlesque performance or the Ziegfeld Girl was meaningful is to focus on a part of cultural life not traditionally privileged for serious study. It is no surprise that in 1981 Lewis A. Erenberg noted that the "cultural importance" of the *Ziegfeld Follies* had not been seriously addressed by scholarship.[55] Erenberg's *Steppin' Out*, his study of New York nightlife, was an influential early model of cultural analysis, the study of how popular practices, such as urban cabaret life, are related to social conflicts and beliefs. Analyses such as Erenberg's have powerfully eroded previous academic distinctions between a "high culture" (sophisticated, aesthetic; for example, Shakespearean productions) and a "lowbrow culture" (superficial, trivial; for example, the *Ziegfeld Follies*) in terms of what these practices actually show us about historical and social changes.

The *Ziegfeld Follies* occupies a curious position even under the old categories of high and low entertainment. Ziegfeld's conscious ideal was the elevation of the "lowly" chorus girl into the realm of upper-class gentility. Even his Anna Held project, biographer Charles Higham explains, originated in his dream "to reject the coarse, vulgar, ugly atmosphere of vaudeville and replace it with glamour, taste, and charm." As Toll comments, however, Ziegfeld himself was seriously committed to superficiality: "All his life [he] had been concerned, indeed consumed, by superficiality in both his personal and professional affairs. He had nothing else. Appearances were his only reality." That very preoccupation with surface, visual appearance, and spectacle makes the Ziegfeld enterprise a valuable case study in the emergence of modern visual culture and its gendered, racialized dimensions. Because the *Follies'* most lavishly constructed spectacles were organized around the display of white female bodies, showcased as ideal commodities, the Ziegfeld enterprise illustrates in a startling way what Teresa de Lauretis calls a technology of gender, widely disseminated in other cultural practices such as film, journalism, and celebrity culture.[56]

The Ziegfeld Girl exemplifies what Michel Foucault calls a deployment of sexuality, a way in which sexuality and the body itself are constructed by social discourses and practices at a particular historical moment. Foucault's scholarship is notoriously indifferent to questions of gender and is highly problematic as a tool of feminist criticism. Nevertheless, citing Foucault we can speak of the Ziegfeld Girl not as a monolithic image but as a knowledge, multiply disseminated and circulated within various kinds of discourses. Moreover, we can understand the implications of the Ziegfeld Girl as known body. The social nuances of Ziegfeld's glorification enterprise suggest the kind of power dynamic Foucault names as the primary modern, Western political force beginning in the eighteenth century: "Through the themes of health, progeny, race, the future of the species, the vitality of the social body, power spoke *of* sexuality and *to* sexuality," he writes. My work on Ziegfeld emerges in the context of the considerable scholarly response to the Foucauldian concept of historicizing sexuality and the body and in particular to Foucault's exhortation to examine "a specific type of discourse on sex, in a specific form of extortion of truth, appearing historically and in specific places." [57]

Along those lines, my attention to the Ziegfeld Girl as a specific historical body is influenced by current feminist concern for the body as the very material of culture rather than its passive object or vessel. The Ziegfeld Girl embodied multiple social contentions, exemplifying one way in which early-twentieth-century concepts of commodification, racial categorization, and nationalism were actually manifest and lived. Her status as fantasy, wish, and cultural projection are inseparable from her status as social, psychic, racial, and biological lived body — not the object or symbol of knowledge but the knowledge itself. I am thinking here of Elizabeth Grosz's eloquent descriptions of the body as a threshold between binary categories of the public and private, cultural and biological, psychic and social, constructed and natural. "The body must be regarded as a site of social, political, cultural, and geographical inscriptions, production, or constitution," Grosz tells us. "The body is not opposed to culture, a resistant throwback to a natural past; it is itself a cultural, *the* cultural product." [58] Using this model of the body, my assumption throughout this book is that the Ziegfeld Girl can be understood as one intersection of major American social issues during a specific era. Her iconography had multiple uses and significations, but she herself was readable text and the embodiment of its topics; indeed, the topics of glamour, racialized nationhood, and showcase heterosexuality could exist only through specific bodies as manifest and understood in practices such as the showgirl.

Far from positing this study as the complete social meanings of the Ziegfeld Girl, I hope it opens up the various and contradictory ways this figure was influential in the past and continues to be mythologized in the present. My primary materials were the contemporary representations of the Ziegfeld Girl, not just her performances onstage but her strong textual life outside the theater as well. These representations—the magazine stories, advertisements, news releases, films—are a field of discourse, a set of contentions and arguments through which the Ziegfeld Girl emerges as an example of wider social concerns.

The Ziegfeld Girl as sexual fantasy is inextricable from the cultural fantasies she embodies and her cultural work as a category of identity. The durability of the Ziegfeld Girl legend, its vigorous ability to outlast the theatrical and showgirl style, suggests a striking nostalgia for a "guaranteed" and knowable sexual/racial body, even if it posits that such a body existed only as need, fantasy, hype. Indeed, the camp and drag queen renditions of this showgirl satirize the impossible project of constructing such an authentic or original body out of theatrical material, feathers, and pearls. The producer and product, Glorifier and Glorified, have apparently incorporated powerful cultural themes and concepts—or, put more accurately, have incorporated troubling questions and unresolved issues into a more palatable package. Imagining this variety of fantasies and desires, we are certainly far from that turn-of-the-century spectator who wanted "the facts of life." But the Anna Held performance was no such "fact," either, and the Ziegfeld enterprise vividly illustrates how such facts are invented.

CHAPTER ONE

Celebrity and Glamour: Anna Held

A Glimpse into the Boudoir

More than a decade before Ziegfeld's Follies Girl appeared on the New York stage, her immediate predecessor made an off-Broadway splash that rippled through theater and pinup girl history. In the 1890s, Florenz Ziegfeld was more interested in the uniqueness of individual stardom than in the production of a brand-name "type." As a publicity stunt for the performer advertised as Parisian chanteuse Anna Held, his first female musical star, Ziegfeld arranged the "news" that she took a daily bath in fresh milk—supposedly one of her scandalous French beauty secrets. To provide evidence for eager journalists, Ziegfeld choreographed what would now be called a media event, with deliveries of milk being timed for the arrival of reporters. The reporters—and by extension, the public—were invited into Held's suite for a glimpse of the luxurious Anna in her creamy bath, a move that invoked both nudity and its occlusion in one brilliant stroke.

The 1896 milk bath incident, perhaps the original American beauty-in-the-bubble-bath image, has become a signature item of Anna Held, included in every biographical sketch and foregrounded in the 1936 film *The Great Ziegfeld*.[1] At its time, the milk bath made titillating headlines for weeks and supposedly started a brief fad, an auspicious beginning for Ziegfeld's aggressive publicity blitz for Anna Held as a daring European performer. "The name of the young woman became as well known in this country as the name of the President," the *New York World* declared a year after her arrival.[2] Less well known, but rumored and often denied, was her previous Polish Jewish identity as Hannale or Annhaline Held, *choristka* of Jacob Adler's Yiddish theater. In her more recent incarnation as the imported Parisian music hall singer, Held starred in a number of musical-comedy hits on Broadway and on tour from 1896 until 1912. Though she never appeared in his *Follies,* Anna Held continued her asso-

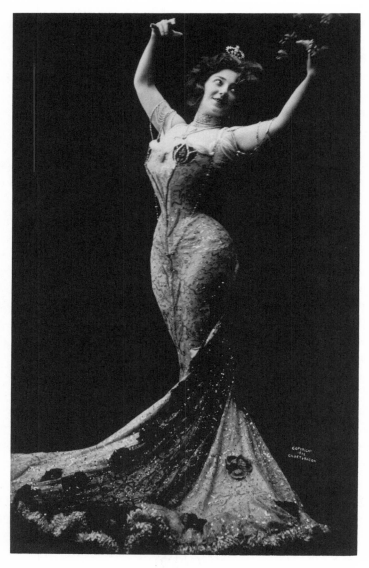

Anna Held, circa 1898. (Billy Rose Theatre Collection, New York
Public Library for the Performing Arts)

ciation with Ziegfeld throughout that period, during which he was her manager, common-law husband, and producer of many of her shows.

More important, Anna Held sustained her status over the years as a particular kind of celebrity, a turn-of-the-century embodiment of how female sexuality could be publicly known and visualized. The milk bath episode—as public relations, legend, and fantasy—suggests the meanings of her body as a tease between sexual knowledge and secrecy, between visibility and imagination. As a herald of the Ziegfeld publicity style, the milk bath stunt also presages the economics and dynamics of the later Ziegfeld Girl promotion. The milk bath media event organized sexual knowledge as class privilege and commodification, the economic luxury of hundreds of bottles of milk. The entire package also promised authenticity—an exposed body, an imported beauty secret.

While the milk bath remained the Anna Held legend par excellence, her later publicity also focused on her famously corseted waist and her notoriously mischievous eyes, all three sensationalized through teasing strategies of concealment and revelation. But the concealment most carefully maintained in her representation was her ethnicity and race: her eastern European origins and her Jewish parentage. Ziegfeld publicists positioned Held as a desirable female heterosexuality precisely through its distance from those identities and through its definition as western European (French beauty secrets) and as class entitlement to certain commodities.

Recent studies of stardom have emphasized its function in cultural debates about meanings of gender and sexuality. Tracing the development of stardom in silent cinema, for example, Richard deCordova uses this approach to develop insights particularly relevant to Anna Held's celebrity. DeCordova describes the star's body and persona within the modern project of "speaking sex," in Foucauldian terms, of making sexuality available as a discourse. The personality of the early film star, he argues, was orchestrated as a series of "secrets," or teases about the "real" person behind the screen image. The ultimate "truth" of the star was his or her sexuality, with sexual scandal being the "primal scene of star discourse."[3]

The Anna Held case illustrates, first, how much cinematic practices of star promotion are indebted to earlier theater practices and, second, the specific historical nature of the star's "secret," in this case, the relationship between racial and sexual knowledge/secrecy. Held's commodification and her circulation as sexual imagery were constituted by issues of authenticity, revelation, and transgression directly linked to her Jewish identity, its occlusion, and its curious status as an "open secret." The "ultimate truth" of Held's stardom was not simply a primal scene or even the body in the milk bath but also a specific cultural scene, European Yiddish vaudeville, positioned as lower, dirtier, and grittier than the upscale Broadway trade, but also more fascinating for its sexual energy.

Anna Held's high-profile discourses on Parisian fashion and beauty tips were the standard entrée for imported female celebrities at the turn of the century, offering the Old World as elegant shop. But for Held, these discourses were also loosely layered strata under which the Old World lurked with its damp, musky secrets. Anna Held's appeal rested within the liminal space between these two Old Worlds, fashionable and filthy. Her music hall comedy, her borderline-risqué song lyrics, and her usage of African American dialect songs link her to the style of Fanny Brice, who would make her name in the *Follies* near the end of Held's career. The Jewishness on which Brice based an entire comic style, however, was exactly what Held had to repress and what became, in effect, the forbidden underside of her desirability.

As all this suggests, Anna Held's marginal position in the Ziegfeld enterprise—her moment previous to the Glorified American Girl—illustrates the exclusion of ethnicity and transgression in the development of the latter. Eventually, Ziegfeld's publicity promises about women and authenticity would lead him away from Anna Held's European exoticism and toward a redefinition of what he would call "native" Americans—that is, toward the Glorified American Girl. Many of Ziegfeld's Follies Girls became, like Anna Held, individual stars whose particular talents and bodies were promoted as unique. But "glorification," the rhetoric assuring a standardized, guaranteed quality, was per se an abstraction and idealization into a recognizable "type." Anna Held's performances, saucy and intimate, in those theaters "so small you could touch her," embodied an earthiness from which the Glorified Girl—particularly the posing, clothes-model *Follies* showgirl—would be removed.

Illusion, Fetish, and the Baffling of Facts

In popular theatrical history, the Ziegfeld Girl has overshadowed Anna Held precisely because the later Ziegfeld pitch for a nationalized Girl was so successful. But the publicity campaign for Anna Held was also, in its time, a nationwide coup. At the peak of her career in the 1900s, journalists referred to "the Anna Held craze," the widespread public fascination for the woman who "couldn't make her eyes behave." Eddie Cantor and David Freedman remember the "craze" lasting for an entire generation, and their account of its commodification reads like a laundry list of fetishes: "There were Anna Held corsets, facial powders, pomades, Anna Held Girls, Anna Held eyes and even Anna Held cigars." [4] Cigars indeed.

Throughout the "craze," New York newspapers gave sensationalized coverage of each publicity stunt for Held (a record-breaking series of kisses, a challenge to an automobile race, purchases of fabulous horses) and carried press releases about her beauty and fashion advice and her various proclamations chiding American women for their prudery ("A leg is a leg, not a leemb," she declared). But newspapers around the country—from Rochester to Toledo to St. Paul and San Francisco— were equally attentive to this Parisian import, especially in the wake of her nationwide tours. [5] She was featured as well in national journals such as *Vogue,* the *Cosmopolitan,* and later the *Green Book.* Even the seriously oriented *New York Times,* openly critical of Held's talents, nevertheless covered her career and personal life thoroughly, giving front-page attention to her supposed betrothal to Ziegfeld in 1897 and later to her filing for divorce from their common-law marriage. [6] After her estrangement from Ziegfeld in 1912, she continued theatrical work in the United States and then in Europe. The regular newspaper updates of her final illness and the accounts of thousands of people at her New York funeral suggest her celebrity was still going strong at her death in 1918.

The professional creation of entertainment personalities was gaining momentum in the United States at the time of Ziegfeld's 1896 debut of Anna Held. Public relations as a business was relatively new in that decade and was primarily associated with the theater. By the time the *Follies* was first produced in 1907, film studios were also becoming savvy about the use of publicity to generate interest in individual players. The concept of Florenz Ziegfeld as "the man who invented women," which I cited in my introduction, is more accurately tied not to the mythic power of a Broadway producer but rather to these machineries creating the public personality and the public body. By the late 1920s, the industrialization of celebrity was complete, including the production of specialized fan magazines and the established professions of press agent and publicist.

This new industry created glamour: not an illusion or abstraction but a real way of thinking and perceiving desire and sexuality. Florenz Ziegfeld did not originate this quality, but he was enormously influential in its proliferation, from Anna Held through the Ziegfeld Girls. Glamour, like voyeurism, requires both visibility and distance, goals of the public relations business in producing insatiable, commodified desires.

Channing Pollock, one of Ziegfeld's publicists, has described his own work in those days in creating client visibility. As Pollock makes clear, image was all, and advertising budgets were slim, so publicists depended on the fake news story. "The fake story became more than part of our job; it was a matching of wits with city editors, and the filling of a demand for news far in excess of the supply," he writes in his memoirs. Explaining the Anna Held milk bath episode, Pollock compares publicists, as "professional liars," with novelists. Novelists, he concedes, "admitted writing fiction, while we had to baffle shrewd investigators pledged to print only facts." The "baffling" with facts marks the beginning of modern public relations as a specialization or perversion of journalism. Like his predecessor P. T. Barnum, Ziegfeld demonstrated that the ideal publicist was a "creator" rather than "purveyor" of news.[7]

The milk bath episode also illustrates the slippery nature of authenticity in the publicity business and the necessary manipulation of distance (between star and fan) that would become important characteristics of the twentieth-century celebrity business. As Joshua Gamson points out in regard to contemporary celebrity sightings, "the celebrity encounter is used to confirm and reconfirm that surfaces have something, in this case someone, beneath them."[8] Thus authentic bottles of milk appeared for Anna Held in time for reporters, who were then granted distanced glimpses of the bath itself. For both glamour and

Anna Held Facial Cream, Anna Held Eyes

Throughout her career with Ziegfeld, Held was publicized specifically as the Parisian tutor of American women on issues of fashion, beauty, and jewelry. The Parisian identification immediately authorized Held's sexuality and desirability. French was "the naughty language" because it was the language of Flaubert, Zola, and Balzac.[12] Paris was home of the wicked *Folies Bergère* and the site of Toulouse-Lautrec's music halls. Theatrical imports, farces with French origins and ribald overtones, were popular in American theaters through the 1890s. Held's music hall precedent was the French singer Yvette Guilbert of the Moulin Rouge, made famous by the paintings of Toulouse-Lautrec, brought to the United States in 1893 by William Hammerstein, and similarly renowned for the eroticism of her songs, even though her impact was never as sustained and nationalized as Held's.

A decade after her debut in the States, Held gained new notoriety in Ziegfeld's 1906 musical *The Parisian Model,* in which she made a number of costume changes onstage, with the chorus girls as her only screen. The published Held memoir claims it was a controversial show, prompting moral condemnations that "made so much publicity . . . that there was a dreadful crush at the box office."[13]

Held's suggestive persona, no matter how risqué, could nevertheless be packaged into previously established mainstream venues. First, celebrity beauty advice had already been institutionalized in American popular journalism. As music hall actresses such as Lillian Russell gained respectability, popular theater became a source of upscale fashion authority. By the 1890s, magazines such as the *Cosmopolitan* regularly carried features on the hair and clothing styles of stage actresses. Second, Held was able to draw on the image of a European aristocracy that, though fictive in her case, was easily established through the connection with fashion. Newspapers ran regular pages on "society in Europe" that included "General Surveys of European Centres of Fashion" as well as interactions with European notables, royal news, or "Personages in Europe Who Interest Americans," as the *New York World* titled their sections.[14] Other European performers with careers in the United States—

Alla Nazimova, Anna Pavlova, Lina Cavalieri, Olga von Hatzfeldt, and Gaby Deslys (who was later overpublicized in a similar way by the Shubert brothers)—likewise were regarded as authorities on dress, cosmetics, and hairstyles.

Anna Held's celebrity authority on beauty is a good example of how such advice produces not just a consciousness of beauty standards but a gender and sexuality as well. Cantor and Freedman's list of "Anna Held corsets, facial powders, pomades, Anna Held Girls, Anna Held eyes" illustrates how the identity and body is conflated with the corset and pomade. Generally, Held's fashion interviews centered on the body as shaped by its clothing: the ways to hide a thin neck, the secrets of using jewelry to accentuate pretty hands, and, most of all, the art of the corset.[15] This extension of the body through costume, and costume as instruction of gender, remained an important dynamic in Ziegfeld's later productions of women stars in the *Follies*.

Granted that corsets were widely advertised by the 1890s, Held's lengthy, spirited interviews on corsetry revel in the details of this intimate clothing, setting up a powerful dynamic of the invisible in relation to the visible, the inner and outer body. In multiple interviews, Held supposedly describes the colors, fabrics, and jeweled hooks of her corsets with affection. Held's voice in these interviews is shamelessly conflated with fashion and society journalism: "The climax of dainty eccentricity has been reached in corsets of rose pink lace lined with pale rose silk. Each corset hook fastens with a ruby."[16] That is, Held's willingness to be associated with corsetry fashion made it possible to attach her image and authority to articles on "How to Lace Tight without Doing Yourself Harm" and the superiority of the more pliable French corsets to their stiffer American equivalents. For several decades after her death, it was widely believed that Held died fairly young, at forty-five, because she had injured her organs with the strong stays, and the story is repeated in print as late as 1964 by Ziegfeld's daughter, Patricia.[17]

The tease of revelation/concealment in the dress/corset discussions is repeated visually in photographs of Held. The top-heavy effect of the powerful corsetry turned her entire body into a fantastic bow tie–shaped vessel, in which her waistline has nearly disappeared and her breasts look enormous. Early commentary about Held in newspaper and journal articles constantly refers to her "perfect little figure" and the famous tiny waist, although this may have been a euphemistic way of referring to her breasts as well. As an acquaintance later remembered, she was "a well-stacked girl."[18] Held's hourglass figure was strikingly similar to those of the burlesque queens, the High Roller Girls who dominated burlesque posters of the era. Unlike those powerful burlesque beauties, however, Anna Held projected exotic delicacy, partly through her diminutive stature and partly through her more genteelly coded poses and gestures in publicity photos.

Held's eroticization of corsetry may seem at odds with the "naughtiness" of her image if tight lacings can mean only inhibition and restriction. But recent studies of fashion have reconsidered the corset as an apparatus of self-consciousness about the body. Confinement in fashion wear has been cited as a sexualizing device, a sign of restraint that acknowledges what unrestrained sexuality means. Other studies situate corsetry as an erotics of visibility to others, a "mapping" of secret parts. Historian Casey Finch points out how the hourglass figure popularized in the nineteenth century replaced the "fertile, belly-centered body," shifting attention away from a woman's reproductive capacity to a more suggestive eroticism of "corsets, crinolines, and bustles"—in short, of secret places with mysterious capacities. As media scholar Jennifer Craik has described clothing of this era, "the corset lurked under the respectable facade of respectability, as a constant reminder of impure thoughts and unconscionable acts."[19]

Held's praises of tight lacing set up a preoccupation with the body's invisible spaces. The volatility of those spaces was guaranteed by the risqué nature of some of her trademark songs: "I Just Can't Make My Eyes Behave" and "I Really Wish I Wasn't but I Am." Because of this defining relationship between body and clothing, Anna Held's expertise on the corset and pomade enabled her expertise on the female body itself. Advertisements and promotions of her shows suggest the appeal of this expertise for a female audience, as is evident in the ad for *The Parisian Model*: "All who see the performance come again and send their mothers, sisters, children, cousins, aunts, and friends." In Held's published memoir, there is also a reference to an audience of "mostly women" at a matinee.[20] When she rolled her huge eyes and sang, "It's Delightful to

Be Married," Anna Held was addressing female heterosexual pleasure in a not-so-circuitous way.

A passage in the Held memoir interprets her fans as a repressed audience eager for release: "Ordinary people loved me. In me, they recognized their secret desires. I helped them to discover their true character, buried under a mound of prohibitions." [21] Yet the very proliferation of Held's image contradicts that what she found in turn-of-the-century America was simply "a mound of prohibitions." Her popularity was very much enabled by understandings of sexuality already in circulation, the inconsistencies rather than the rigidities of a strict puritanist code. If anything, Held's turn-of-the-century popularity suggests, along the lines of Foucault's thoughts on the "repressive hypothesis," the instabilities of American "Victorian" heterosexuality.

Historians of American sexuality usually point out a widening gap in the 1890s between the sexes in terms of sexual knowledge, especially for the middle to upper classes that made up Held's audiences. Particularly in urban areas, access to female prostitutes was increasingly common, and the high rates of male venereal diseases in such areas are startling—perhaps as high as 80 percent of all men in New York City in the first years of this century. The chasm between expectations of female purity and male sexual experience may have been "a major area of tension in turn-of-the-century sexual life," historians John D'Emilio and Estelle B. Freedman claim. [22]

The tension was exacerbated by the ways in which sexuality was being addressed for female audiences through conservative, middle-class practices: "marital advice" literature, reform work that acknowledged the problem of prostitution, and the growing proliferation of work by scientists claiming to classify sexualities. Anna Held was related to these practices indirectly, through a rhetoric that firmly placed her within standardized white, heterosexual, middle-class formulas at the same moment she was offered to the public as the sexualized Parisian.

Her stardom was constituted by a bundle of spoken secrets—the beauty bath, the teasing glimpses of a body radically redesigned by corsetry—but also by more domestic "secrets" circulated as middle-class desires. In its more obvious tactics, the Held publicity often presented a traditional woman, a domestic expert who gave advice about chafing dishes and menus as well as advice on how to flirt with a parasol. She heartily recommended marriage for women, not just in the saucy song but also in serious interviews probably directed at the growing number of educated women who were not choosing marriage: "I do not believe that anything has so broadening an effect upon the feminine character, mentally, morally, and every other way, as a husband and the responsibilities of the married state."[23] Ironically, she and Ziegfeld never legally married (perhaps because of her fear of his financial recklessness), but what the biographies call an "unofficial ceremony" took place in 1897, and she was referred to thereafter as Mrs. Florenz Ziegfeld in her private life. This play of the racy and the respectable would be the dynamic of Ziegfeld's later productions of female stars.

Further evidence of the traditionalist strategy is found in the great number of antisuffragist statements Held supposedly made, a stand very different from that of her friend Lillian Russell (who always spoke on behalf of the woman's vote). In a 1910 interview, Held's instructional tone about fashion is directly linked to politics, with the complaint that proper feminine clothing would be absurd at the voting polls: "I can't think of anyone going to vote with curls and laces and strings of pearls. . . . I don't care at all who is president if the lace on my bodice is put on right."[24] Anna Held's articulation of sexuality, then, was made possible through both an aggressive expertise of the body as mapped/specularized by fashion and through domestic, nonthreatening discourses of the "lady," with curls and laces and strings of pearls, who is careful not to make a spectacle of herself at the voting polls. However, the convergence of these strategies around vision and visibility itself, the famous "Anna Held eyes," foregrounds how the issue of "speaking sex" is interlocked with speaking gender and race as well.

The emphasis on Anna's eyes reached its apotheosis in her 1906 song "I Just Can't Make My Eyes Behave," a whimsical tribute to the flirtatiousness of her "bad brown eyes" that beckon men to "play." Five years later, newspapers and magazines were still running commentary on Held and women's eyes as instruments of flirtation. Her memoir calls it Anna's "triumph as woman and as artist."[25] If the naughty eyes are the counterpart of the corsetry instruction—the emphasis on what is visible—they are also an interesting emphasis on female vision in relation to sexuality.

On the one hand, the function of the eyes is reversed in some of these fashion journalism discourses, so that what they look like ("There Are Eyes and Eyes: Are Yours the Pretty Kind?") is more important than looking. On the other hand, the sexual ideology of vision gets reversed as well, especially in many references to Held. Eyes that "misbehave" are active and can even be aggressive. To some extent, this flip-flops the cultural assignation of power to the masculine gaze. Misbehavior, after all, connotes transgression, in this case a double transgression of sexual mores and traditional female demeanor. Publicity photographs of Anna frequently have her posing in ways that emphasize her eyes, winking or widening them for the camera in unsubtle come-ons.

Anna Held's "misbehaving eyes" may have served not just as instruction in flirtation but also as recognition of a greater female agency and independence than had been possible in earlier times. Recent cultural studies have directed attention to the active female gaze of the shopper, tourist, museum-goer, and audience member at the turn of the century.[26] The split nature of the "eye" craze—setting up female eyes as both objects and agents—may be symptomatic of this larger social movement, in which white women were both given more mobility and access to public space but also positioned, especially through advertising, theater musicals, and the new art of cinema, as sights themselves.

Anna Held's celebrity illustrates the racial explicitness of this exoticized female eye, the constitution of its Caucasian whiteness precisely through its association with an exotic Other. "It is the Oriental eye that dominates New York now at the height of the season," claims a 1907 news story. The accompanying photographs show that turn-of-the-century Orientalism was also at the height of its season; Anna Held, along with actresses Lina Cavalieri and Alla Nazimova, Europeans who were similarly regarded as experts on Continental elegance, are the models of this ideal eye. This appropriation of European actresses makes sense in the logic of commodification, in which the mysterious element of the Orient can be obtained through a costly purchase. "The Oriental eye is the eye with a riddle in its depths," the story explains, advising that kohl can give the illusion of the fashionable almond eye, although "a very small supply costs from $1 to $2."[27] The desirable image is a white woman, not an Asian woman, but the desirability depends on an association with another race.

If this practice was an acceptable way to "speak sex"—the Oriental "riddle" implying a sexual knowledge—it was also, then, a way to speak race. The sexuality performed by Anna Held was constituted by racial hybridity: middle-class whiteness crossed with a marginal, possibly threatening Other. The terms of this construction—Anna Held as both white European and racially exotic—are even more complicated in their origins, erasures, and redefinitions.

Choristka, Chanteuse, Coon Shouter

Anna Held's identity as a European "lady" was the key to marketing her as the secret of white sexuality and to marketing attractive female sexuality as white. Fitting into this fashionable nook meant, for Held, the circumventing of her far less fashionable ethnicity. As one Ziegfeld biographer discreetly put it, her Parisian origin was ascertained "for professional reasons." Held was born in Warsaw, Poland; her father was French Jewish, and her mother, Polish Catholic. The family emigrated to France when Anna was a child. Held's published memoir emphasizes that Anna had been brought up as a Catholic, but biographer Charles Higham claims she converted from Judaism to Catholicism at the time of her first marriage in France.[28] Arriving in New York during the decade when Jewish immigration was particularly intense and not especially welcome, Anna Held arrived with a secret cultural past.

Held's European career had actually begun in Yiddish theater under the tutelage of its foremost director, Jacob Adler. According to his biography, Adler discovered Hannale or Annhaline Held among the choristkas at his Prince's Street theater in London. Adler immediately trained her for starring roles, and she continued in Yiddish theater as a headliner until she moved into European vaudeville, where she was equally acclaimed. By the time Ziegfeld saw her in Paris in 1896, her previous Yiddish work had vanished in her new identity as the Parisian chanteuse. Years later, when Adler appeared at Held's dressing room to visit, she refused to see him.[29] Sexual scandal may be the "primal scene" of stardom, but in the early twentieth century, racial scandal was the more repressed scene, and perhaps the more unspeakable.

Held's covert Jewish background, refashioned as Parisian chic, is situated curiously in the racial inflections of what "sexiness" would eventually mean. Anxiety about racial whiteness during this era was crossed with the fascination for racial and exotic Otherness, as seen in the popularity of the "Oriental eye" and exotic beauties Cavalieri and Nazimova. The figure of the Egyptian, South Seas, or Turkish beauty continued to be featured throughout the *Follies* era, into the 1930s.

This fascination perhaps accounts for the odd open secret of Held's Jewishness. Newspaper articles occasionally identified her "Polish Jewish parentage" or more obliquely referred to the "clever race" to which she owed her success.[30] Newspaper cartoons of the era often caricatured Ziegfeld himself (actually of German Lutheran heritage) as Jewish, probably conflating his German name and the Jewishness of many other Broadway producers of the time. Ironically, then, the rumors of Anna Held's origins may have merged with incorrect assumptions about her producer/common-law husband. Held's public responses consistently emphasized her mother's Catholicism and, even more so, her fictional Parisian birthplace, an origin that also conveniently associated her with both fashion and sexual chic. When she reapplied for a French passport in 1915, she reported to the press that only then "she learned from friends of her family that she really was born in Warsaw."[31]

Yet transgression and scandal—the association with the darker races and lower classes—were in fact deployed by Anna Held and by other mainstream Broadway entertainments during this era in less direct ways. Transgressive performances by women often employed the grotesque as an articulation of sexuality—that is, of parallel "lower-body" activity. Vaudeville's Eva Tanguay, for instance, the "I Don't Care" girl of the early 1900s, appeared onstage in disheveled costumes and shocking white tights associated with burlesque theater. Later, Sophie Tucker combined class transgression with Jewish comedy to enact the "last of the red-hot Mamas." These performers originated in marginal, lower-class theaters but gradually were popularized in upscale Broadway revues. The vulgarity of these performances as "low-other" is a clue to their hybridity, to use the term familiarized by Peter Stallybrass and Allon White; they functioned on the borderline between acceptable and unacceptable public articulations of female sexuality and, in doing so, made the struggle and the articulation possible.[32]

The grotesque performance tradition in which Anna Held often participated was coon shouting. The period 1890–1910 saw the vast popularization of coon songs and coon shouting, a derogatory form of African American songs performed primarily by white women, often but not necessarily in high-yellow blackface. Coon songs used vulgar imitations of black dialect, and their lyrics were explicitly racist. Popular coon shouters such as May Irwin had Broadway musical shows of their own (*The Swell Miss Fitzwell,* 1897). Comic Jewish female singers had a special niche in coon shouting. As Pamela Brown's work on this phenomenon reveals, coon songs were the linchpin between minstrelsy and Yiddish musical theater. They were central to the work of Sophie Tucker, Nora Bayes, and Fanny Brice, all of whom performed them later for Ziegfeld's *Follies.* Coon shouters used comedy, minstrelsy traditions, and poses of female sexual aggression to appeal to "audiences struggling with race-consciousness and Victorian old-world moralism," as Brown puts it.[33] The popularization of coon shouting by Jewish women singers compounds the racial cross-performance here, bringing two "low-other" associations into gentrification on mainstream stages.

Though Anna Held herself did not perform in blackface, she did utilize African American entertainment styles and coon songs, many of which marked her best-known comic performances. Her published memoir includes a description of one of these, a cakewalk and the coon song "I Want Dem Presents Back," sung in a Parisian accent so that the "novelty was all the more daring." The mise-en-scène of this 1897 song and dance routine is particularly startling. On the stage backdrop for her song were painted giant bars of sheet music, the notes cut out so that "the woolly head of a Negro" protruded from each, the memoir reports: "thirty-three black noggins swayed, rolling the whites of their eyes, to the rhythm of the song."[34]

Coon songs specifically used grotesque imagery either in the lyrics themselves or in the cover art of music sheets, often suggesting hybrids of black people and animals or of babies and adults. Held's unique costume for "I Want Dem Presents Back" is notable. Her upper torso rose from a wicker basket fastened around her waist, from which the mannequin of a black man's torso sprouted forward. The effect was Anna in a sedan chair or litter "being carried by a graying Negro, bent almost in two," even though the legs seen by the audience, in wide striped

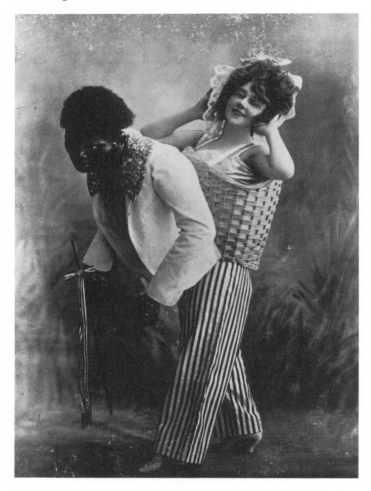

Anna Held and "trick" puppet costume for the coon song "I Want Dem Presents Back," 1897. (Billy Rose Theatre Collection, New York Public Library for the Performing Arts)

trousers, were her own. "This act was so successful that Flo quickly had it copyrighted," Held's memoir notes, but in fact this trick costume can be seen in photos of other revues of the era as well.[35]

The confounding effect, however, is not simply the "trick" of the disappearing legs but the haunting image that Anna has sprung a "Siamese twin," joined at the waist, and that the white showgirl has suddenly put on display her full meaning as acceptable public body created by the co-presence of the unacceptable black one. Held's face and head are framed by her hands, emphasizing the pleasing nature of her own image to herself and others, and she smiles confidently into the camera. But this pleasing public body is tethered to its dark other self, which, in contrast, is pointed away from the camera's gaze, the head tilted downward, the bent figure the carrier of the upright one. The referent here is perhaps Beauty and the Beast — the dark mannequin as the beast of burden for Beauty — but the physical symbiosis of this image complicates it further. The placement of the dark mannequin just below Anna's waist is explicitly sexual, for one thing, as if her sexuality, what cannot be expressed by the cute showgirl in ribbons and curls, is projected onto the racial Other. Yet there is no denying this Other as interior, "always already" part of whiteness rather than outside it, to use Eric Lott's argument.[36] Lott's work on blackface is relevant here because Held's wearing of the mannequin is an equivalent of the black mask, the mixed sign of identification and abhorrence, attraction and contempt.

Glamour always implies the relationship of distance, which is necessary for fetishization, so particular prohibitions constitute that distance at a specific historical moment. The image of Anna Held singing a coon song in a French accent suggests these strong social measurements of distance: she invokes the low-other but also disavows it, while the invocation of a Parisian expertise of the body reinforces a hierarchy of desirability. Her own participation in a socially designated low-other — eastern European Jewishness — and the status of this identification as a badly kept secret illustrates the complexity of stardom and celebrity at a given time, the circuitous and contradictory relations between knowledge and desire.

Toward the end of the Held-Ziegfeld relationship, cultural pressures for images of an "American" girl in musical theater may finally have worked against Held's European allure, especially in light of her debated Jewish identity. Ziegfeld's involvement with his female stars, younger and fresher than Held, was no secret, even from Held. Biographers agree that the most important of these women was Lillian Lorraine, the leggy showgirl who was Ziegfeld's most influential mistress and possibly

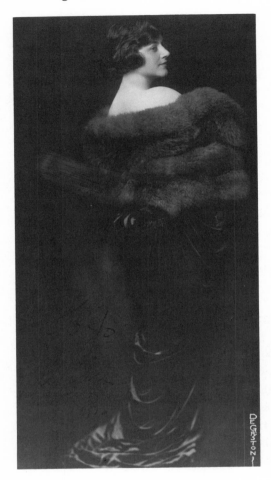

Lillian Lorraine, who replaced Anna Held as Ziegfeld's foremost star and who would become the prototype clothes model/Ziegfeld Girl. (Billy Rose Theatre Collection, New York Public Library for the Performing Arts)

the inspiration for a tall, American-style revue girl. At one point, Ziegfeld actually established Lorraine in an apartment in the same building in which he was living with Held. Ziegfeld's amorous adventures and cavalier financial risks were finally too much for Held, who left him in 1912, continuing her theatrical work on her own.

Ziegfeld's taste in women at that point had moved decidedly away from dark exoticism and toward fair-haired Nordic types. When he married the titian-haired Billie Burke in 1914, she was at the height of her stage reputation as "the little English girl." Burke had actually been born in Baltimore but had done some work on English stages, and there is more than a little Anglophilic affection in the moniker. Unlike the sensuous Held, Billie was marketed as the wholesome girl next door. The publicity machines that had constructed Anna Held as "sultry" and "mischievous" produced the new wife as "sweet," "serene," and "our own." In 1918 she was able to pose for *Theatre Magazine* as a hybrid angel–Red Cross nurse with a demure earnestness that would have been impossible for the sexy Anna Held; she was also able to be entirely distanced from the taint of "foreignness." "Know Why You Never Saw a Hun in Billie Burke's Plays?" a 1918 headline asked. "No Germans," says the Billie Burke persona in what sounds like a manufactured interview. "I don't even want to see one in the 'extra' ranks."[37] In 1916, *Ladies World* presented a Billie Burke cutout doll with dancing frocks fit for little girls' middle-class fantasies, a venue wholly unsuitable for Held's more dramatically sexualized body. The shift in bodies that we see in these transactions around Ziegfeld's women is indicative of the larger project and agenda of the showgirl. Although both Ziegfeld wives were publicized and promoted as prototypes and ideals, Burke was specifically tracked as the Anglicized beauty that the Ziegfeld enterprise would "glorify" from World War I into the Depression.

Coda: Authenticity and Reproduction

The published memoir *Anna Held and Flo Ziegfeld* concludes with a chapter by Held's daughter, Liane Carrera, who describes her mother's melodramatic deathbed scene in which Held was supposedly declared dead but then came back to life for a few hours for one "last curtain call."[38] Indeed, Anna Held's resurrections in public representation constitute a second career.

In 1987, Ginger Rogers received a remarkable letter from the ninety-two-year-old Carrera, asking if Rogers would be interested in producing a Broadway play about Held's life. For Carrera it was one of many unsuccessful efforts to restore Anna Held to the public domain and equalize her fame with that of the Ziegfeld Girl. Carrera died the following year, and the play was never produced, but the event is a signature of Anna

Held's life as public figurehood, a life heavily invested—successfully by Ziegfeld, unsuccessfully by Carrera—in its representation.

The 1936 film *The Great Ziegfeld* represents Held melodramatically, as the tragic woman cast aside, a stepping-stone to Ziegfeld's artistic ambition. In her last scene, she tearfully fakes happiness in a congratulatory phone call to Ziegfeld after his marriage to Burke, then presumably succumbs to death by broken heart. Refusing to accept this as the final public scene for her mother, Carrera energetically wrote and rewrote her mother's story, as evidenced in a number of unpublished manuscripts in the archives at the New York Public Library for the Performing Arts. The book she published in 1979, *Anna Held and Flo Ziegfeld,* is supposedly a translation of her mother's memoirs but suspiciously duplicates much material in the other manuscripts. She also opened the tiny Anna Held Museum, first in Manhattan and then in San Jacinto, California, displaying Held's clothing and other belongings. At the end of the tour, visitors could glimpse through curtains a life-size mannequin of Held at her dressing table. "And now to our pièce de résistance," the museum visitors guide proclaimed. "Anna Held herself at her dressing table in her bedroom. Just look at every minute detail."[39]

When Held first came to the United States with Ziegfeld, she gave to her first husband, Maximo Carrera, full custody of the infant Liana. As early as 1906, rumors of Anna Held's French "adopted" daughter circulated in American newspaper reports. When Maximo Carrera died in 1908, Liane was brought to the States and secretly shuttled in and out of the Ziegfeld household until the papers got so suspicious that reporters had to be invited in for the story—though Ziegfeld and Held lied about Liane's age. "For a tragic actress, it might be all right to be the mother of an adolescent girl," Held's memoir notes. "But would not such a discovery be damaging to the career of a titillating music-hall star whom the public wanted to think of as 'naughty?'"[40]

To the contrary, publicity about a hidden child and "a past" in France proved to be one more sexual secret come to light, and the news about Liane was soon exploited rather than repressed. The same play of concealment/revelation that devised the milk bath and corsetry stories begins to come into the daughter stories in 1908. (Is there really a daughter? Will she be put into a show? Does she know her mother's reputation?)

Liane's arrival in the States was nearly as publicized as Anna's. "Anna Held's Daughter Has Never Seen Mother Onstage, Girl Comes to NY," headlines blared. The narrator of *Anna Held and Flo Ziegfeld*—that is, either Held or Carerra—claims that Ziegfeld relentlessly set up Liane as the counterspectacle to Anna, a publicity gimmick focusing on the "secret" child, by having Liane come to performances and sit in a prominent seat. But whatever conflation of voices or authors it represents, *Anna Held* is replete with confirmations of Held as her own best publicist, and it suggests a different reading altogether: that Held herself was happy to use Liane as a hint of a scandalous past.

Anna Held and Flo Ziegfeld powerfully conveys Held as an ambitious actress who fully participated in and encouraged public relations. I have been describing Held's careful construction by Ziegfeld's publicity agents, but I am not at all implying a passivity on the part of Held. The memoir documents her full cooperation with publicists and her enthusiasm for continuous press coverage. After she left Ziegfeld, Held continued to generate publicity on her own, including a wonderfully wild story that she visited a movie set in France and single-handedly shot a runaway tiger.[41] Until her illness, she managed her own career in American vaudeville and in European theaters. In the last years of her life, she even tried work in the cinema, starring in Oliver Morosco's *Madame la Presidente* (1916). It was kindly reviewed as revealing that "Anna Held 'joost can't make' her eyes behave for the movies, either," a full twenty years after her dramatic American debut. Even on her deathbed, Held was apparently thinking of her public and composed a fittingly melodramatic good-bye for the press that, citing a French Catholic saint, adds one final confirmation of her identity as *not* Jewish or Polish: "It is the last curtain. I have lived, and I will hold out to the last—it is the spirit of Joan of Arc and the spirit of my parentage—the indomitable French."[42] The spirit may have been saintly, but it was also practical. Held's estate at the time of her death was worth nearly a quarter of a million dollars, a stunning contrast to the impoverished condition of Ziegfeld when he died fourteen years later.

Liane Carrera was herself on the vaudeville stage by 1917 but never attained anything close to her mother's popularity. Even before her mother's death, she used the stage name Anna Held Jr. and later proceeded to reproduce her mother in other ways—the manuscripts, the museum, the attempt at a Broadway play. The masculine touch of the name—becoming Junior—seems appropriate for the daughter of such a phallic, fetishized mother. Perhaps Carrera was making a reclamation against the powerful forces of the Ziegfeld century, which eventually cast Anna Held as a minor player instead of a featured star.

Considering she had been virtually abandoned by her mother until she was thirteen, Carrera's obsession to make Held appear again also continues the process of concealment and revelation that marked Held's career, with the pièce de résistance being the mannequin in the boudoir, the mother who will not disappear. The 1980s tourists in San Jacinto who were coaxed to glimpse into Anna Held's dressing room and "look at every detail" provide a fitting coda to Held's public life, which in turn brings together issues of celebrity, fetishization, and the discourse of white female heterosexuality in the United States at the turn of the century.

At one point during my research, I reached into an envelope at the Billy Rose Theatre Collection and, to my astonishment, pulled out a small leatherbound booklet, Anna Held's handwritten address book. Having it in my hands was for a moment shocking, as if I had touched flesh—like the guest in *Wuthering Heights* who reaches through the broken window glass and touches the ghostly hand on the other side. The hundreds of pages of clippings about Held had worked for me—this was celebrity, and I had touched its surface and found something "real" underneath. But my account here of Held's public representation is no attempt to reclaim a "real" Anna Held, whatever that might be, but rather an effort to describe a strategy. The organization of Held's public image—the focus on fashion as an expertise of sexuality, and the implicit racial hybridities of that sexualization—prefaces the tactics that would be used by the Ziegfeld enterprise for decades.

CHAPTER TWO

Chorus Girls, New Women, True Bodies

A 1909 story in a New York Hearst newspaper claimed with great ado that a "chorus girl factory" had opened in Manhattan to train those with potential. "Do you want to be a showgirl? Stand before the mirror to see whether you possess all of the requirements," the story instructs.[1] The newspaper story is actually about the opening of a dancing school on Broadway, but the factory reference obliquely acknowledges the working-class appeal of chorus girl life and—perhaps with unintended irony—how popular images of women had become factory processed by 1909. According to some 1904 newspaper estimates, there were ten thousand unemployed chorus girls in New York City and sixty thousand chorus girls for every opening position.[2] The truth is that real factory life—the garment trades—was far more likely to be the destiny of working-class women during this decade in New York City. But here is the promise of far more interesting work, as well as an assumption that the applicant is willing to be factory processed if a certain social mirror measures her as suitable for "show."

Through the manipulations of glamour, Anna Held had been rendered "suitable for show" as a hybrid of racial and cultural exoticism. Her niche, however, was the individuality of stardom; she was "the comet of the century's end" whose uniqueness made her valuable property. In Ziegfeld's *Follies* of 1910, Anna Held—by then in her thirties—appeared as a more distanced representation, in a projection of film footage emitted from a special-effects blazing comet. She was more directly displaced in the *Follies* by blond, leggy Lillian Lorraine, who had already displaced her in the romantic and personal life of Ziegfeld. Lorraine appropriated Held's signature foaming-bath imagery in the *Follies* of 1909 by singing "Nothing but a Bubble" in a soapy tub. The progression from Anna Held to Lillian Lorraine is the progression in Ziegfeld's work toward an "American" rather than a European beauty ideal. Eventually,

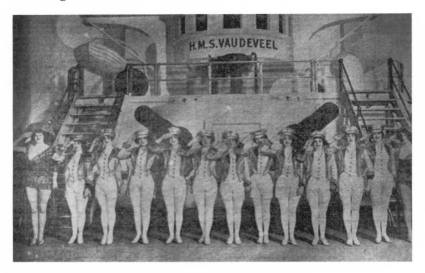

Ziegfeld Follies showgirl lineup, 1912. (Billy Rose Theatre Collection, New York Public Library for the Performing Arts)

Ziegfeld's women stars such as Lillian Lorraine were packaged both as unique properties and as standardized or "guaranteed" images—chorus girls "glorified" by the Ziegfeld factory.

In this chapter I describe how the Ziegfeld Girl emerged as a type and ideal from a theater world and a popular culture that idolized the chorus girl in the first few decades of this century. The serious engines of this idolization—and frivolization—are apparent in the industrial image of the "chorus girl factory": women as paid workers and women as productions of consumer culture. The chorus girl as publicly visible working woman could connote, during the Ziegfeld era, a number of positions ranging from the prostitute to the more ambiguous, transitional figure of the New Woman, one of the icons of female independence in the first few decades of this century. The larger issues here are the growing visibility of women in the public sphere and redefinitions of gender that involved questions of sexuality as well: the knowable or "true" female body.

Cult of the Chorus Girl

Although gender roles are constantly in the process of construction and invention, cultural historians describe the Ziegfeld era, the first three decades of the twentieth century, as a particularly significant one. The undermining of Victorian prudery and traditional roles for women was well under way by the 1890s as an ethic of leisure gradually emerged as an acceptable strand of modern life. This ethic encouraged the pleasures of leisurely shopping and consumption, as well as the pastimes of dancing, movies, and amusement parks. These new spaces and occasions for leisure time marked the closing of sex-segregated Victorianism and the beginnings of what historian Kathy Peiss calls "the affirmation of heterosociality."[3] The availability of these new heterosocial spaces affected popular conceptions of proper public behavior for women and men. Mixed-sex public amusements such as nightclubs and afternoon dance cafés, in combination with the fast, suggestive new dance crazes, profoundly eroded traditional concepts of gentility, modesty, and courtliness in relations between the sexes. Describing this new mixed-sex scene, Lewis A. Erenberg emphasizes that the gender concept most clearly in decline was the Victorian stereotype of True Womanhood—the assumption that there was an essential womanly nature that was pure, nurturing, homebound, and demure.[4]

Such an assumption had always been less than monolithic in nineteenth-century America, as I suggested in the previous chapter in my discussion of the popularity of Anna Held.[5] But even as a social ideal, the selfless, domestic image of True Womanhood would not survive the urbanization, industrialization, and commercialization apparent in the first decades of the new century. The discourses of feminism, progressive reform, and suffragism during this era further scrambled older female gender codes. Although these political movements were undertaken by a small minority, the reverberations were much wider because they coincided with these other social changes affecting traditional ideas about gender and family.

In the gradual shift away from Victorian ideas of womanhood, the chorus girl figure was both marginalized, as lower-class and associated with prostitution, and centralized, as a popular, nonthreatening challenge to traditional ideas about female modesty and the place of women outside the home. As historians have persuasively documented, the chorus girl at the turn of the century became a symbol of liberation and independence — "the modern girl," as Erenberg puts it, but also a central figure in "tensions that women and men found with the new informal personality, the lowering of barriers, and the subsequent inability to discern confidently which women were 'true' and which were not."[6] In some ways, then, this figure made palatable a number of gender characteristics associated with the progressive New Woman during this era — independence, mobility, professionalization, and a delay of marriage.

From the turn of the century well into the 1920s, the chorus girl was not merely a theatrical position but also a mythology and prototype, a recurrent character in American fiction, film, journalism, and the tabloids. The prominence of actresses such as Lillian Russell who "rose from the chorus" romanticized chorus life as an opportunity and an adventure. Costumes became scantier over this period, and the revue shows in particular became more daring in their flashes of legs and bosoms. The title of the P. G. Wodehouse and Guy Bolton memoir, *Bring On the Girls!*, named after a well-known 1922 *Follies* number, accurately sums up the popular enthusiasm. Describing their own experiences in musical theater from 1906 through the 1930s, Wodehouse and Bolton emphasize that in the repetitive stream of so-so theatrical musical comedies, the energetic choruses were often the saving grace of the show. Significantly, for a book named after and dedicated to these performers, the chorines themselves are mostly faceless, nameless background entities behind the male world of production. Ziegfeld is part of the world described in this book, and his demand about a particular comedienne encapsulates the tone: " 'Make her young and cute,' he said. 'I hate women comics.' "[7] To the contrary, multiple sources provide evidence that Fanny Brice was one of Ziegfeld's favorite people, but the wisecrack remembered by Wodehouse and Bolton characterizes the bottom line of the "bring-on-the-girls" mentality.

The turn-of-the-century chorus girls, in their sedate gowns and bustles, hardly seem to match the racy stories accumulating around them in newspaper columns, but the ambiance — bring on the girls! —

was similar to that of later, leggy chorus cuties. What Robert C. Allen calls "feminized spectacle" had become common on theatrical stages in the United States since the 1860s; burlesque, ballet, and equestrian drama exemplified strategies for containing the "social transgressiveness" of the female body on display. By the 1890s, choruses of European opera were being mimicked in American popular-culture musicals, so chorus girls were used extensively on vaudeville circuits, in musical theater, and in revue shows. The chorus girl was thus a legitimate theatrical position, even if designated as lower-class and only marginally respectable. Located on "the fringe of the dramatic world," explains theater historian Benjamin McArthur, the chorus girl "needed good looks, a fair voice, knowledge of a few dance steps, and perhaps most important, a fashionable dress for the job interview." [8]

The *Cosmopolitan, Munsey's,* and other magazines often featured stories about chorus girls, and the *Green Book* magazine followed suit in the second decade of the new century.[9] Feature journalism was especially fond of this theatrical figure. A *Variety* columnist in 1916 noted how "the papers teem with her — all the good old stuff about the johnnies and the automobiles and the farewells at the railroad stations." [10] Given William Randolph Hearst's marriage to a former showgirl and his longtime association with another one, it is not surprising that the Hearst newspapers in the first decades of this century gleefully represented the cult of the chorus girl — the stage-door johnnies and other admirers — as an exciting space of transgressive relationships. The chorus girl stories were hyperbolized with photographs and provocative headlines: "May Ask Court to Stop Chorus Girl's Wedding," "Showgirl Miss Virginia Lee Engaged to Eleven Men." Competing newspapers followed suit. Stories of chorus girls' involvements with society men — elopements, vampings, divorces, and romances — were carried regularly. Headlines such as "Danced Barefoot into His Heart: Chorus Girl's Pink Tootsie-Wootsies Won Bibbins, a Princeton Student," were not feature stories but front-page news.[11]

The *New York World* theater critic Roy L. McCardell, a significant publicizer of chorus girl life, sensationalized the chorus girl with headlines and metaphors suggesting her commodity value: "It has been a feverish week in the chorus girl market," "Beauty Market for Broadway's Summer Shows Closes at $1000 a Girl." He also shamelessly mystified the working life of this figure. In the lifestyle he paints, the young women spend four afternoon hours of rehearsal and four hours of performance in the evening, but they are not always onstage for those hours. "The rest of the time they are gossiping, eating candy, doing fancy work or just taking it easy." The chorus girl represented by McCardell is primarily a consumer, not only of hats and dresses but also of taxi rides and dinners paid for by male admirers.[12]

McCardell's novel *Conversations of a Chorus Girl* was a national bestseller in 1903 and was imitated by others, so titles such as Madge Merton's *Confessions of a Chorus Girl* (1903), Grace White's *Fallen by the Wayside, or a Chorus Girl's Luck* (1907), and Frank Deshan's *Chorus Girls I Have Known* (1905) became commonplace in popular fiction. These fictions often portrayed chorus girls as clean-cut young women enjoying their independence, dating college boys, and remaining "good girls" throughout. But such texts also illustrate an underlying nervousness about sexuality, respectability, and relations between the sexes, issues for which the chorine was clearly a litmus test.

The heroine of *Confessions of a Chorus Girl,* for example, has run away from a convent school to join a musical show that travels the East Coast. Thus the story is framed in a rejection of several traditional values—religion, sex segregation, celibacy, modesty—in favor of mobility, bodily exhibition, and, most of all, mixed-sex social life. In every town, college boys treat Madge and her chorine colleagues to dinners full of alcohol and cigarettes. This is not courtship of any kind but "fun"—a heterosexual space still so new that the silly conversations are included line by line, as examples of "racy" ways a mixed-sex crowd could talk.[13] As opposed to the private, sacramental confession back at the convent, this confessional voice is very much a public deployment, in Foucault's sense, a voice that assumes a listener who requires it. While her narrative uses a playfully subversive voice, it is far from subversive or threatening to the culture pruriently interested in a recounting of these details.

McCardell's *Conversations of a Chorus Girl* is similarly structured as a series of vignettes tantalizing the reader with behind-the-scenes information: "I'm from one of the best families of Altoona, Pa., and my mother would die if she knew I wore tights on the road." But McCardell's focus is the chorus girl relationship with men as an exchange of goods—companionship in return for jewelry, champagne, dinner at

Rector's. McCardell explicitly links commodities being sold onstage with the selling of this racy new female character. In one episode, "a friend in the wine business" offers the chorus girl a case of brand-name champagne for each time she and her fellow chorines sneak the brand name into the show in a little ditty about "bashful girls." At the conclusion of the song, "one of the bashful girls would turn cartwheels, while the other would stand on one foot and hold the other up in the air, playing on it like as if [sic] it was a guitar." [14] With a knowing wink to the reader, the chorus girl later stands up "the wine friend" in a great moral huff, making clear that the raised skirts and splayed legs are—at least in this comic representation—simply part of her job.

In this respect, the chorus girl prototype illustrates the careful middle-class management of sexuality that Peter Bailey has described regarding the Victorian barmaid in Great Britain in the 1890s. The barmaid was one of the attractions of the public house, supposedly a "good" girl but suggestively visible in her place behind the counter with other commodities. Bailey describes her "parasexuality . . . sexuality that is deployed but contained, carefully channeled rather than fully discharged." The barmaid made the tease of illicit sex imaginable: "She was respectable, yes; she was the girl whom a chap might just marry, by jove; she was also the girl who just might . . . without one having to marry her" (Bailey's ellipses). [15]

The female body as knowable and reliable—that is, with a respectable class, racial, and sexual identity—had become an issue with the growing visibility of women in the public sphere. In a Times Square scenario at the turn of the century, the would-be female consumer might actually be a commodity herself: "The woman would linger at a shop window and wait for a man to approach her with the formulaic 'Anything doing tonight, dearie?' " [16] By the turn of the century, new public, urban locales—the department store, the arcade, the museum, the movie theater—were available for the middle-class white woman who had previously been circumscribed by the privacy of the home. The result was a new social figure, neither a "woman of the streets" nor the traditional, homebound wife. However, the growing presence of "nice" women in public places, at shop windows and in theaters and parks, elicited a great deal of commentary by social reformers and vice squads anxious to read sexuality in daily public scenes. [17]

The chorus girl as "working girl" was closely associated with prostitution. References by reviewers and other journalists to the perpetual stage-door johnnies imply that chorus girls, like prostitutes, provided pleasurable company for the male subculture that was distinctly visible in parts of New York, a subculture in which class lines were regularly transgressed in pursuit of illicit sex.[18] The proximity of the chorus girl to the streetwalker was a literal one in that the Times Square area had always been surrounded by a red-light district. Broadway in particular was noted for its upscale street trade, and some of the best nearby restaurants, such as Rector's, provided private chambers for after-dinner dalliances. Chorus girls were often categorized with kept women as consumers and commodities in this market. An often repeated line from a 1906 Weber and Fields revue sums up the nuances: "A chorus girl is asked if she ever found a pearl in an oyster; she replies, 'No, but I got a diamond from a lobster over in Rector's last night.' "[19]

Avery Hopwood's long-running, immensely popular 1919 Broadway play *Gold Diggers*—which coined this phrase—represented this version of the chorine who, in blatant exchanges of companionship for hats and jewelry, approximated prostitution. "All women of the theater are chiselers, parasites, or—as we called them—gold diggers," one male character explains. Among themselves, the chorus girls in this comedy discuss how much they should "give" in return for gifts, because, as one points out, "either you work the men, or the men work you."[20]

These references to work and working girls suggest that the great cultural interest in the chorus girl was not simply a prurient one but also a deflection of the problems incurred in the growing presence of women in the workforce. During an era in which sexual appeal was increasingly being defined in terms of youth, the chorus girl redefined women's work as sex ("young and cute"). In this fantasy, working women could be taken less seriously, as less likely to upset traditional sex and gender roles in the workplace. The visibility of women in the professions, in reform work, and in politics rose sharply from the 1890s to 1930. Statistics may be simplistic as indexes of the social and public scene of that era, but they chart profound changes. In the period between 1890 and 1920, the increase of women in professional careers rose a startling 226 percent. These careers included not just traditional ones such as teaching but business and law as well. Between 1890 and 1900, the presence

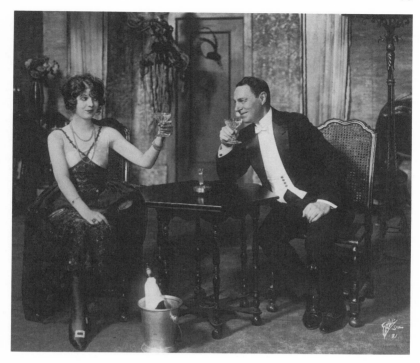

Ziegfeld star Ina Claire in Avery Hopwood's *Gold Diggers* (1919). (Billy Rose Theatre Collection, New York Public Library for the Performing Arts)

of women in graduating college classes rose from 25 to 40 percent. By 1915, nearly half of the female college graduates were professionally employed. Less educated women also moved out of strictly domestic work and into service work as office help, salesclerks, and waitresses.[21]

The actual social effects of this new and growing workforce are difficult to gauge. On the one hand, workplaces for most women, the factory and the clerical office, reinforced rather than subverted traditional gender roles; women workers were paid poorly and remained in lower positions within the business. On the other hand, even if nondomestic work did not wholly transform women's political and social positionings, it nevertheless complicated one level of their cultural interaction. Accounts of working-class women in factories, for example, show that they experienced a social life there previously not possible when their work had remained primarily within the home.[22]

The chorus girl emerges at the intersection of these issues, a romanticization of "women's work" which avoids questions of authority and education and which further connects women to issues of appearance and decor. The chorus girl also represented a fantasy solution to the real problems of working-woman life in that her narrative supposedly ends safely in marriage to a special member of the audience. The upper-class man could comfortably marry "down" in this case because the new currency of "fun" could compensate for the slippage in class. The chorus girl's marriage to the millionaire was the apotheosis of this mythology, as supposedly occurred with the original Floradora Sextet in 1900.

While the Avery Hopwood play was still onstage, a 1921 *Theatre Magazine* essay on chorus girls posed the question, "Is the lady of the ensemble a 'gold digger' or is she an 'actress?'" Is the chorus girl an exploiter of men or a professional woman? Threat or thespian? Predictably, the essay concludes that she is not necessarily either: she is impossible to explain except that "we should sadly miss her if she did not cheer us with her opening chorus."[23]

The cheer she brought no doubt worked on several levels in placating gender tensions. The refusal to define the chorus girl as either gold digger or actress is the refusal to confront the contradictions of what modernity and its promises of freedom actually meant to women in this era.[24] The supposed freedom and independence of the chorus girl masked the actual economic dependency of most women on men. She might share or use some of the language of the ambiguous New Woman—"independence," "freedom," "cleverness"—but it was easy to distinguish the chorine from serious feminists or suffragists. And, finally, as birth control and discourses of female sexual pleasure became available in the 1920s, the chorus girl's sexuality and sexual knowledge were all the more significant as part of her appeal "on show."

The sensationalized world of theater and women "on show" was highly publicized in the 1906 Stanford White murder and the subsequent, drawn-out trial of the socially prominent Harry K. Thaw. One of the earliest celebrity criminal trials, the case was dominated by the image of Thaw's wife, Evelyn Nesbit, as former showgirl, model, media personality, and alleged victim of a previous rape by White. As White's great-granddaughter put it, his "murder was an iconic event at the juncture of centuries," Victorian hypocrisy meeting modern sensationalism.[25] Nesbit as "former showgirl" continued, on a higher-class scale, the performance of her own sexuality as spectacle, object of speculation and mixed desires. The body of the chorus girl, accessible to the college boy or businessman, was thus vividly represented as both desirable and punished, object of awe and violence, romanticized and raped.

Wet Swimsuits

In short, the cult of the chorus girl was well in place when Ziegfeld launched his first *Follies* revue in 1907. His over-the-top innovations would become his signature: fifty chorus girls instead of the usual dozen or two and an upscale venue—the New York Theater roof's Jardin de Paris, combining the popular roof garden entertainment format with the hint of Parisian sophistication for a respectable middle- to upper-class audience. To distinguish his Follies Girl from chorus girls of other revues and shows, Ziegfeld actually put her name on the program; even in the first *Follies,* the dancers are specified, so that we know "a showy girl" is played by Viola Kossard, and "the showiest girl" by Lois Bard.

The Anna Held Girls of this first revue, though named for the well-established singer, referred in their routines less to European glamour than to the carefree American chorus girls of the Hearst newspapers and McCardell's columns, fun-loving modern women in smart gowns and fashionable accessories. Moreover, the most publicized skit and image from this early revue suggests the link between the frivolity of the chorus girl and the larger issues of knowable and suitable female modernity. Ziegfeld's first Follies Girls may have been named for Anna Held but were Gibson Girls in their primary advertising gimmick and theatrical staging, associated with both a specifically American image and a non-threatening representation of modern female independence.

The Gibson Girl was perhaps the most palatable and popular icon of the era's controversial New Woman. The latter was an especially ambivalent, though powerful, rhetorical and visual strategy. This "new" modern woman was educated, knowledgeable about birth control, associated with feminism, and present in the workforce in record numbers. The New Woman was also a shorthand representation of far more contradictory issues and attitudes, ranging from conservative eugenics to radical reformism to women's athletics. While some of her political implications place the New Woman at a considerable distance from the Ziegfeld Girl, these figures as cultural icons also overlap in telling ways. Far from operating as a frivolous alternative to the serious New Woman, the Ziegfeld Girl from the start used the other image as a way to embody a version of modern womanhood that was suitable for show.

The progressive debutantes sketched by Charles Dana Gibson and his imitators (Howard Chandler Christy, J. C. Leyendecker, and James Montgomery Flagg) were cloned as plucky and athletic, though always elegant and feminine, New Women. These female images implicitly promised that the demands of the modern New Woman would not exceed comfortable bicycling and tennis clothes. These images also promised she would be white, fashionable, and from old money.[26] The Christy Girl illustrates this mixed bundle of social issues in the 1906 picture book *The American Girl As Seen and Portrayed by Howard Chandler Christy*. Free of "narrow-minded conventionalism," the accompanying text tells us, she believes in outdoor exercise, hygiene, and health. More telling, her assets are "education and race." She claims "English cousins" and some French passion, but she is utterly distinct from "the young peasant woman, who, bundle in hand and kerchief on head, makes her awkward, blundering way amid the throng of emigrants that has been landed in one of our great cities and gazes stupidly upon the wonders of the New World."[27] The modern American Girl, then, was specifically a racial creation, marked through her opposing, negative image by both visibility and vision: her fashionable appearance (no immigrant kerchiefs on head) and her better ability to see (and purchase) the wonders of the New World.

Theatricalizations of Christy Girls and Gibson Girls were not unusual when Ziegfeld staged the latter as part of his first *Follies* in 1907. "But as Mr. Gibson's creations represent very distinct types of American girls, it needed only judicious selection on Manager Florenz Ziegfeld's part to exactly reproduce them," as one reviewer explained.[28] Ziegfeld had previously secured a reputation for serving up classy but racy female images; the previous year, Anna Held had boldly changed clothes onstage, shielded only by the warm bodies of chorus girls, in his production of *The Parisian Model*. Not surprisingly, Ziegfeld's Gibson Girl did not "exactly reproduce" Gibson's but looked ahead to how the American pinup tradition and *Sports Illustrated* would prefer American girls: in swimsuits.

In the summer of 1907, Ziegfeld had secured the rights to use the Gibson image for his *Follies*, which would in turn be advertised through Gibson bathing features in the *New York World*. On the *Follies'* stage, Gibson Girls forsook their habitual athletic wear or evening gowns and in their song pleaded for Mr. Gibson to get them out of their long elegant dresses and to paint them instead "with dimpled knees . . . and plenty of rounded limb." [29] The *World's* promotion for this *Follies* attraction was not subtle in its depictions of who could and who could not be a Gibson Bathing Girl. One feature story quoted the song from the *Follies* skit: "There's a peach, a peach of a Gibson bathing girl," with a sketch of the Follies Girl and an insert cartoon of a chubby woman in a bathing suit, captioned, "This variety of peach not wanted." [30]

The blatant specification of desirable and undesirable bodies suggests that even this early in the Ziegfeld revue history, the Follies Girl literally embodied fashion and social ideals. In the long-range Ziegfeld project, varieties of female bodies "wanted" and "not wanted" would be further specified through the conflation of body and clothing, with desirability packaged as a unified fashion, class, and race. This conflation is clearly at work in these first Gibson Girls/Follies Girls as bodies suitable for certain clothing: "Mr. Ziegfeld has had the time of his life picking out tall girls who can also wear bathing suits gracefully," the same feature tells us, "but the statuesque beauties have finally been found, and Mr. Ziegfeld proudly announces them as the most attractive show girls ever presented to public view." In the 1909 *Follies*, the swimsuit/body on display went a step further, with the women in swimsuits well doused with water, providing "an opportunity for the wet suits to cling revealingly to the fine figures of the girls" à la wet T-shirt contests much later in the century. [31] This bolder definition of the female body functioned conservatively in the long run, in delineating an "authentic" female body at a moment when the authenticity of that body and "true" womanhood had become destabilized.

If the Gibson/Christy Girl was the New Woman at her most sexually and racially palatable, her most threatening versions were suffragists and, more indirectly, lesbians represented in grotesque satirical cartoons of the era. The caricatures of suffragists as hideous hags suggest the significance of physical appearance in women's political issues at this time; feminism could be mocked because it was embodied, at least in popular imagination, by women who dared to be in the public eye but were not pleasing to look at. Thus in a 1917 essay in *Vanity Fair,* a ridiculous claim about favoring a showgirl to political activist Emma Goldman illustrates how showgirls functioned as a preferred visible sign of supposedly liberated modern womanhood. Goldman, as working-class immigrant, is certainly the Bad New Woman, whereas the theatrical star fits into the spectrum of spunky Gibson-Girlesque New Womanhood: "I prefer pretty girls, smart girls, clever girls, vivacious girls, lively girls. I would rather look at [theatrical star] Muriel Martin for five minutes than at Emma Goldman for five hours," claims the male writer.[32] In other representations of the era, the New Woman is perniciously portrayed as vampire and siren, or as Salome, less a political creature than a mythical one in fin de siècle "portraits of evil." [33] In the wake of Oscar Wilde's play, Salome clones had become popular, controversial theatrical attractions, writhing and dancing suggestively, a parody of which was also included in the first *Follies.* This very range of images and politics suggests that, as opposed to the warm knowability of True Womanhood, this New Woman was much more diffuse and contentious as an ideological construction and even as an image.

As opposed to the widely publicized Gibson Bathing Girl, thornier versions of New Women, especially suffragists, were prime material for *Follies* satire. "That Ragtime Suffragette" in the 1913 *Follies* keeps her husband waiting at home for dinner while she shouts for votes in the street:

> Hagging and nagging in politics,
> That Ragtime Suffragette!
> She's no household pet!
> While her husband's waiting home to dine,
> She is ragging up and down the line.[34]

The mainstream suffragist movement was actually just as bourgeois as the *Follies,* but its comic potential was clearly its threat to domesticity. "The Vampire," another song in the *Follies* that year, similarly addresses the current "vamp" figure as the doom of unknowing husbands: "I bet the man who wrote *The Vampire* certn'ly must 'ave known my wife."[35] In a 1919 magazine article, the Ziegfeld persona conflates these songs and images, vampire and suffragette, in characterizing the Follies Girl as the ideal "type" of woman. "A lot of girls make the mistake of trying to imitate the vampire type. . . . My advice to them is to forget it! The vampire is not a popular household pet."[36] This quotation reappears in more recent accounts of the Ziegfeld Girl as the wholesome alternative to more threatening "vamp" images of women early in the century. As I point out in Chapter 4, however, the more significant threatening female images referenced in this particular article are the Jewish and immigrant women who could not possibly be considered attractive, or even American, in 1919.

The Follies Girl, spunky and gorgeous but eager to be domesticized, was in fact the household pet who was neither frightening nor political. Describing her loveliness, Ziegfeld's preferred public relations term was "pulchritude." Eddie Cantor and David Freedman recount that Ziegfeld's favorite three words were " 'Glorification — Femininity — and Pulchritude.' If he saw the word 'Pulchritude' in a press agent's story he didn't read any further. He knew it was O.K."[37] The three linked terms are openly nostalgic for Victorian True Womanhood. In the satirical comedy numbers of the *Follies,* the chorus girls appropriated daring "modern" identities marked by outrageous costumes and special effects: as aviators, baseball players, taxicabs, Jazz Babies, and automobile drivers. Nevertheless, the overall implication was that the most modern and daring of all female occupations was that of Follies Girl herself, true femininity and pulchritude. This was the gist of the immensely popular Ziegfeld production *Sally,* the 1920 vehicle for Ziegfeld Girl par excellence Marilyn Miller. Sally rises from dishwasher to *Follies* star, marries a millionaire, and simply vanishes in bubbles of chiffon and taffeta. The *Sally* narrative sweetly sanitizes the themes of Hopwood's satirical *Gold Diggers* of the previous year. Unlike Hopwood's scheming chorus girls, Sally progresses from one naturalized female state to another: kitchen, stage, marriage, and exit from the public eye, presumably to a more upscale kitchen.

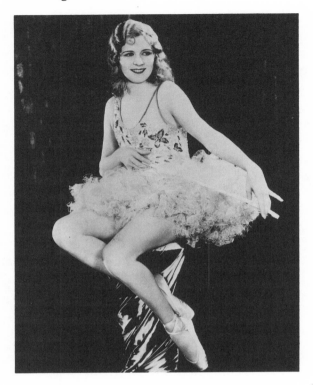

Marilyn Miller, high-profile Ziegfeld Girl and star of
Sally. (Billy Rose Theatre Collection, New York Public
Library for the Performing Arts)

Generally, then, the gender questions of progressive modern womanhood were answered with comedy, specularization, and play in the *Ziegfeld Follies;* the New Woman was visible and knowable in her airplane
or automobile or in her materialization as good-natured Sally. Part of
her knowability was her familiarity as "American" — that is, white, Prot-
estant, with English cousins. In the larger picture, though, it was not
simply True Womanhood but the concept of a "true" female body that
was undermined during the Ziegfeld era. The more unsettling question of female visibility during this era was the sexual question: the
growing visibility of homosexuality. The figure of the New Woman was

linked to new ways of talking about sexuality as well as about gender. The rhetorical position of the Ziegfeld Girl as a true or "guaranteed" female/heterosexual body is thus connected to that era's cultural and medical discourses concerned with sexual differences, categories, and identifications.

New Women and True Bodies: Yama Yama

The handsome book jacket of Richard and Paulette Ziegfeld's 1993 coffee-table opus *The Ziegfeld Touch* can be read as an example of how the New Woman, with her ambiguous connotations, circulates as a cultural subtext that is at once far removed from and yet directly implicated in the figure of the Ziegfeld Girl. The jacket shows one of the more genuinely talented Ziegfeld Girls, dancer Bessie McCoy, in her Yama Yama costume —a fanciful Pierrot pajama. In 1908 the well-known novelist and Hearst reporter Richard Harding Davis fell in love with McCoy during her Yama Yama dance in a Broadway musical comedy. Theater lore claims that when McCoy took her Yama Yama dance to the *Follies* in 1911, Davis watched her from the same seat during every performance for a year.

Davis, his popular imperialist novels now virtually unread, comes down to us in cultural history as the man who invented Hearst's war in Cuba and as the man who squired the Gibson Girl. A friend of Gibson, the handsome Davis was the model for the suave, attentive American man at the Gibson Girl's side. In 1912 Davis finally obtained a divorce from his wife, painter Cecil Clark, so that he could marry McCoy. The divorce and remarriage were widely publicized, merging two exciting popular mythologies: Davis's glamorous life as dashing reporter and the showgirl's glamorous destiny of marrying a distinguished personage from the first row.

The story of the former wife was far less publicized. Early in their courtship, Davis apparently idealized Cecil Clark as the new American Girl, the version of the New Woman who populated his own novels. Cecil Clark was a lover of sports and animals, a rugged traveler, and independent professional artist. She was apparently very similar to Davis's fictional heroines, all spunky comrades with slim, boyish figures and brave blue eyes. "An excellent rider and a standout billiards player, she could have been a model for the tomboy Hope Langham in [Davis's popular novel] *Soldiers of Fortune*. . . . Like Hope, she loved to do the unconventional thing," Davis's 1992 biographer Arthur Lubow points out.[38] Clark insisted on an unconventional marriage: a platonic one of friendship, autonomy, and intellectual pursuit, which lasted for over a decade.

Clark finished a single portrait of Davis, Lubow tells us, which "is rough and unaccomplished compared to her paintings of women, including some striking full-length portraits of women in masculine attire." She enjoyed intellectual conversations with men but "reserved her deepest friendship for women."[39] For the last twenty years of her life, still calling herself Mrs. Richard Harding Davis, she lived with her secretary-companion, Frederica Poett.

The word "lesbian" does not appear in the Lubow biography. My concern here, moreover, is not biographical truth about Clark's life or even the language of her self-identity but rather her position in representation, which turns out to be the vanishing point, a figure almost indiscernible near the horizon. Like the boyish girls in Richard Harding Davis's now-forgotten novels, Cecil Clark is what has been excised from popular representation in favor of Bessie McCoy. Cultural fondness and nostalgia for the Ziegfeld Girl—the glossy coffee-table book published more than sixty years after the close of the *Follies*—displaces that era's more ambiguous, less accessible figure: the New Woman in her more threatening apparitions, from independent intellectual to woman-identified artist, inclined toward the woman in masculine dress.

Yet showgirl McCoy and the less visible Clark pose similar problems in the articulations of heterosexuality in that era. McCoy's hallmark Yama Yama dance, according to contemporary reviewers, was "a wild, fantastic, headlong dance—the dance of a crazy king's clown, half girl, half wild boy," accompanied by her song "in a husky, boylike voice."[40] For Davis, this was part of her appeal, and perhaps not surprisingly, it was the appeal of Clark as well. Up until their marriages, Cecil Clark and Bessie McCoy could equally have encapsulated the spunky, independent New Girl, the more respectable one as the artist and equestrian, the other as the crazily costumed dancer, each with her own career.

But Clark's refusal to engage in traditional heterosexuality keeps her in a kind of Gibson-Girlesque moment, as equitable companion, throughout her marriage. In contrast, McCoy's motherhood and marriage transform her into a tired female stereotype in biographical accounts. As Lubow notes, in his final years Davis was delighted to have a little daughter by McCoy but regretted the loss of Clark. "[Clark's] distance, her coolness, her autonomy—the very qualities that alienated him during the marriage—undoubtedly seemed more attractive now that he was tied to a woman who was hysterically jealous and totally dependent."[41] Davis died of a heart attack just four years after this second marriage. Bessie McCoy went back to the stage, and Cecil Clark continued a successful career in painting, both their lives temporarily interrupted by versions of marriage.

Like the nonthreatening, ever romantic Gibson Girl, Davis's heroines with "boyish" figures are hopeful fantasies that the transition to new gender roles would be easy—that women, if treated equally, will turn out to be good pals, perhaps not so different from men. But this fantasy could not magically transcend the organization of traditional heterosexuality. The split of Davis's desires and needs between Clark and McCoy reveals the vicissitudes of this fantasy for men. For some heterosexual women, desire may similarly have been split between the independent career and traditional family life. Bessie McCoy went back to Broadway after Davis's death, but she continued to give interviews that emphasized her domesticity and motherhood. "But of course they'll laugh. And say, what does the Yama Yama girl know about babies?" she chirps in one such story.[42]

What indeed? On the cover of *The Ziegfeld Touch*, Bessie is theatrically posed on the cusp of a giant, frowning, artificial half-moon, one of the extravagant Joseph Urban props used to showcase the Ziegfeld Girls. A playful fantasy, she seems wholly unconnected to biology, certainly not to motherhood or to monthly female cycles, given the obvious artificiality (and masculinity) of the crepe moon. In her billowy, clownlike, oversized pajamas, she is a woman pretending to be something else, borrowing some props that temporarily obscure gender.

To that extent, the Yama Yama performance disrupted bodily categories in the same way as did the performance of male imitator Florenze Tempest, who was "Our American Boy" in the *Follies* from 1910 to 1914. Tempest could have been read in nonthreatening ways, says Martha

Banta, as "the girl next door having a bit of fun in her brother's clothes." But when Tempest appears in drag with a "girlfriend" or when "she" sings of her love for a man while she is cross-dressed, the semiotics are more complex. "Tempest is a kind of sexual Mobius strip," Banta suggests, "a female, dressed as a man, who sings of 'her' desire to have a boyfriend." [43] If the "boyish" New Woman worked as a fantasy that was not actually viable with heterosexual life, we can understand the performances of Tempest and the Yama Yama Girl as similar fantasies not tied down to biology or other categorical ways of understanding the body. [44]

One could claim that, given the threat of changing roles for women in the Ziegfeld era and the growing acknowledgment of lesbianism, Tempest and the Yama Yama Girl are simply denials and fetishizations of the female body itself, similar to the more obvious fetishizations of women on the Ziegfeld stage: the elaborate costumings of the showgirls as windmills, flowers, battleships, or lightbulbs. All these costumes and performances, however, also suggest the complicated way that heterosexuality was staged as a category for the Ziegfeld audience.

Until the late 1920s, the word "heterosexuality" meant either bisexuality or "perverse" attraction to the opposite sex. [45] A concept of sexual normalcy and a person such as the heterosexual could exist only when categories of perverted sexuality and the homosexual existed in tandem. Before these classifications came into being, devoted same-sex relationships, for men and women alike, were accepted in the continuums of friendship in various ways. [46] In the first decade of the century, public dissemination of the writings of sexologists Richard von Krafft-Ebing and Havelock Ellis had an impact in the United States on popular ideas about such relations. The focus of their writings was not so much the nature of the same-sex relationship as the status or classification of a certain body, the "inverted" body marked by gender characteristics of the opposite sex. The metaphors of this discourse posited an "intermediate" sex, a "Third Sex," "the man trapped in a woman's body." Because our culture places such stock in masculinity, it is not surprising that cultural recognition of a differently marked male body existed even before the medical categorizations. Recent work by George Chauncey documents how the male "fairy" figure was visible and named in urban New York public culture long before it emerged as a medical category. The public presence of the fairy, he claims, was a shaping influence on what would be posited as normal masculinity.[47]

The visibility of the lesbian as an intelligible figure prior to her medical categorization is more difficult to gauge, given socially acceptable practices ranging from romantic female friendship to the Boston marriage, that is, a discreet domestic arrangement.[48] Yet the category of the gender-inverted woman seems to have been acknowledged rapidly in this country following the availability of Krafft-Ebing's and Ellis's writings. While analyzing lesbianism as a physical condition, pathological and congenital, they also specifically linked it to the familiar social figure of the progressive, "masculinized" woman and to that slippery social figure, the New Woman.

These early sexologists were particularly preoccupied with questions of visibility, the literal public appearance and behavior of women, especially those who took on traditionally masculine roles (women of "high intellectual ability," women who smoked cigarettes) and masculinized dress. A biological determinist, Krafft-Ebing categorized "types" of gender-inverted women by degrees of their masculine physiologies, which he then linked to their styles of clothing. Visibility was very much at stake here. "Careful observation among the ladies of large cities soon convinces one that homosexuality is by no means a rarity," he claims. Ellis, far less deterministic, likewise linked the inverted female to "masculine" dress and behavior of the New Woman but insisted that she may not be so obviously marked; her only "masculine element" may be her aggressive attraction to women and her disdain of men.[49]

By insisting that lesbians may appear and behave in traditionally feminine ways, Ellis perhaps provided the more disturbing evidence of the New Woman as a social threat, her perversion utterly undetectable to the unsuspecting eye.[50] Their work was widely disseminated and eventually influenced popular perceptions. Lillian Faderman points out that as late as 1908, magazines carried innocent short stories and poems about women and schoolgirls sharing kisses, embraces, and passionate proclamations of love. Twenty years later, such fiction would have been written and read by most people as demonstrations of disease and degeneration.[51]

The sexual argument provided antifeminists with powerful "scientific" evidence against progressive women as unnatural and anarchistic women-who-would-be-male.[52] The point is that the end of True Womanhood accompanied the questioning of other kinds of categories, not just of acceptable behavior but of sexuality as well. By the 1920s, many people could no longer assume that the female body itself was a knowable, monolithic entity. The visible fair sex could embody other sexualities, not obviously seen and certainly threatening to the status quo.

As a lesbian visibility emerged, it was not entirely censured. The medical discourses of classification, far from shutting down homosexual identity and community, made possible preliminary political and self identifications. On one level, the concept of "gender inversion" led to feminist protest against the artifices of gender itself. Some feminists in the first two decades of the century, responding to Krafft-Ebing, deliberately took on male clothing as a political statement. On another level, available knowledge about a lesbian sexuality made it possible for individuals to name a desire.[53] By this time, too, sexologists began to move away from the theory of "inversion" to suggest "homosexual object choice." A detailed lesbian history of this era is still forthcoming, but self-conscious lesbian identification, specifically sexual, certainly resulted in the formation of lesbian communities by the 1920s, such as those in Greenwich Village and in Harlem; other historians have accumulated evidence that such communities existed in other urban centers as well.

For some groups, this was a deliberate flaunting of what was still, for the public majority, a diseased condition. Lesbians of this era who did not have access to such communities no doubt internalized the pathological characterization or denied their desire. In sophisticated circles, however, lesbianism may have been an exotically acceptable identity. "I only became a Lez because I needed the publicity," Tallulah Bankhead once told Louise Brooks, explaining that "in the '20s and '30s, a Lesbian was tops in desirability, especially with a girlfriend as a side dish." Brooks herself lived for a while with Peggy Fears, who was, she claims, "a lesbian legend, running through the *Follies* beauties like the well-known dose of salts. Every man in New York was jealous of her conquests."[54]

Louise Brooks's claims about lesbian activity, including her own, fluctuated throughout her lifetime, as her biographer points out, but they suggest the growing status of lesbianism as public knowledge during the Ziegfeld period. This status was by no means stable or evenly distrib- uted. Awareness of lesbianism in the 1920s seemed to vary with location, class, and education, so that women's magazines could no longer run schoolgirl romance stories, but show business circles were perhaps titil- lated by this other kind of sexuality. Even here, variable stakes were in- volved. As one more recent critic points out, Louise Brooks and Tallulah Bankhead could afford a lesbian reputation in a way that more main- stream actresses with lesbian inclinations—Greta Garbo and Marlene Dietrich—could not.[55] In terms of visibility on Broadway in particular, three plays with explicitly lesbian characters or themes appeared briefly in the 1920s: Shalom Asch's *God of Vengeance* in 1922 and William Hurl- but's *Sin of Sins* and Edouard Bourdet's *The Captive,* both in 1926. Knowl- edge about lesbianism was probably limited for the average person in the 1920s, but considering the furor created by the plays, especially *The Captive,* female homosexuality had to have been at least acknowledged as a category or identity in some public way.[56]

A number of more recent studies show that the growing visibility of homosexuality in the 1920s shaped efforts to define heterosexuality more clearly, through strategies ranging from consumerism to the "compan- ionate," sexually fulfilling marriage.[57] On the one hand, the high-profile Ziegfeld Girl can be understood as one of these apparatuses reassur- ing a visible, knowable female heterosexuality. On the other hand, the tease of an exotic lesbianism in connection with this showgirl may well have been one of the more submerged pleasures of spectatorship. De- spite the public relations imagery of the "lady" and her elegant stage appearance, the Ziegfeld Girl was nevertheless part of the "liberated" showgirl continuum that glamorized a busy, prominent career (albeit it a short one) for a single woman. Moreover, stage images of linked female bodies in syncopated rhythms, often scantily clothed, may have suggested scandalous possibilities that were in turn quickly recontained by the discourses of bourgeois niceness and male desire—the Ziegfeld oscillation between the racy and the respectable. Some social scandals, especially the ones involving millionaire boyfriends, played well in Zieg- feld public relations; the gold digger notoriety of Peggy Hopkins Joyce was a primary attraction of Ziegfeld's shows in 1917 and 1918. But the

Ziegfeld enterprise aimed to shut down more disruptive images of its Girls, from backstage brawls to addictions; if their romances with Peggy Fears were New York rumors, these stories remained far away from fan magazines and more public forums.

In building a top-shelf entertainment venue with "high-quality" Girls, Ziegfeld skirted issues of modern female independence and sexual freedoms through two major mainstreaming tactics. First, Ziegfeld re-located the romanticized figure of the chorus girl within the codes of avant-garde fashion, merging showgirl and fashion model as a popular model of gender, race, and sexuality. Second, in specifying his showgirl as the Glorified American Girl, he called on the prevailing nationalist rhetoric of an "American race," specifically white and northern Euro-pean, with vested interests in the status quo. In the following two chapters I explore how these strategies operated to secure the Zieg-feld "trademark," the brand-name body that supposedly "guaranteed" a sexuality, a race, and a gender role that were knowable and reliable.

CHAPTER THREE

Costume and Choreography: Fashioning a Body

Given the association of the chorus girl with consumable pleasures and even prostitution, Ziegfeld situated the Follies Girls at a more bourgeois intersection of the body and consumerism: fashion. The transitional element between the turn-of-the-century Broadway chorus girl and the brand-name Ziegfeld showgirl was clothes modeling. The American theatrical world had long worked in collusion with the fashion industry to promote styles and accessories, and the Ziegfeld revue borrowed extensively from this tradition. As early as 1910, the Ziegfeld shows got attention for outstanding costumes; in 1915, this aspect of the show was accelerated with the hiring of fashion designer Lady Duff Gordon, well known as the upscale couturier Lucile, and her models. "The beauties of the chorus and of the specialties must be beautifully clad," Ziegfeld said in a 1915 interview, "else their beauty is wasted or at least discounted." [1] The Ziegfeld revues thus merged entertainment spectacle with display-window commodification and in the process merged costume and Girl into an upscale identity.

J. Brooks Atkinson, drama critic for the *New York Times,* characterized the reputation of the early Follies productions as fairly risqué or "a little sporty." By the 1920s, according to this writer, the Ziegfeld productions had become "eminently respectable and patronized by the best people." [2] In another review, Atkinson specifically linked reputation and class ("the best people") to the *Follies'* chorus girls. The Ziegfeld shows, he claimed, were responsible for "redeeming 'chorus girl' from a term of opprobrium" because Ziegfeld "endows [chorus girls] with the style and the poise of good breeding that make for illusion as they decorate the stage." [3] If "good breeding" can be "endowed" as an "illusion," this gets to the heart of the Ziegfeld enterprise, the mystifying practices of fashion and of public relations.

The association of the Ziegfeld Girls with upscale costuming brought a class and status to the *Follies* that distinguished them from other revues. As early as 1895, American consumers had become literate in the new discourse of corporate advertising that relied on familiarity, iconicity, brand name, and the "guarantee." [4] Like other current brand-name products (Ivory Soap, Elgin watches, Mrs. Winslow's Soothing Syrup), the Ziegfeld showgirl became associated with a "guarantee" of high quality fashion. A laudatory 1915 newspaper article sums up this identity in its headline: "Ziegfeld Trade-Mark Asset to Chorus Girl: Means Beauty, Youth, Animation, Stage Sparkle, and Knack of Wearing Clothes Chic-ly [*sic*]." [5] The latter "knack" was often cited in Ziegfeld rhetoric as an important element in Ziegfeld "processing." "I have taken girls from other shows who didn't give the impression of great pulchritude," one Ziegfeld interview attests, "and when they had been properly gowned they were quite wonderful." [6]

Beginning with the costumes for Anna Held, Ziegfeld banked on the allure of expensive authenticity, not just the illusion of onstage glitter and elegance but the use of genuine silks and real jewels in performances. The Ziegfeld standard for high quality was famous for including apparel not even seen by the audience: Irish linen petticoats and silk bloomers. Anna Held's corsets for her stage shows were studded with rubies. Lillian Lorraine's stockings for the 1910 *Follies* cost $275; one of her costumes for the same show cost $2,500. A 1919 Ziegfeld press release has his loyal chorus girls proclaiming that only the costliest material goes into their costumes, for "only in shoddy chorus girl shows would girls be forced to wear 'cotton tights and $2 shoes. There are chorus girls and chorus girls.' " [7] As I suggested in Chapter 2, this class distinction and the obsession for authenticity worked to guarantee "true bodies" in Ziegfeldian image making, a stabilization of both gender and sexuality.

The centrality of fashion in the Ziegfeld enterprise can be seen in the one Ziegfeld *Follies* production extant on film and accessible to video audiences: the grand finale of *Glorifying the American Girl,* the 1929 film produced by Ziegfeld. The heroine of *Glorifying the American Girl* is first seen in a department store selling sheet music by singing it. At the end of the film, in her glorified state on the Ziegfeld stage, she has moved from representation of a commodity to its embodiment, encased in a tall, sequined headdress and set on a pedestal in a surreal display case of other fantastic living mannequins. A row of chorus girls kicks and sparkles in the foreground, while tall, frozen, gowned women pose in the background. The effect is a performance taking place in a department store, and the dynamics of display and commodification are precisely the mode of "glorification" here.

The identification of the Ziegfeld Girl as clothes model was so prevalent that, ten years after the *Follies* folded, John Robert Powers of the well-known modeling agency felt the need to distinguish his brandname model from the Ziegfeld Girl. The subtitle of his book, *The Powers Girls: The Story of Models and Modeling and the Natural Steps by Which Attractive Girls Are Created,* suggests the continuum of his agenda with that of Ziegfeld's in the Pygmalion-like creation of women. Distancing his model from the Ziegfeld Girl, he points out that the latter "was regarded, for the most part, with lifted eyebrows," whereas the Powers Girl "is often a society girl herself, graduate of a fashionable finishing school, a popular debutante."[8] Although the agenda here is a class distinction, hinting at the chorus girl's more questionable origins and associations, the defensiveness of this argument suggests how seriously the Ziegfeld Girl had actually made a mark as "class."

The Ziegfeld stage-as-department-store, with chorus girls graduated into mannequins, is perhaps the apotheosis of modern entertainment as consumerism. In the first decade of the century, the institution of the nightclub linked the consumption of food and drink to consumption of the show.[9] This practice had been firmly established by 1915 when Ziegfeld opened a club version of the *Follies,* his rooftop *Frolic* shows. While the audience was set up for drinking and dining at tables, the chorus spectacles on display suggested other commodities. In the first *Frolic,* chorus girls paraded in their sumptuous gowns on a runway, a modeling device often used in department store fashion events at that time. In the *Frolic* version, the runway was made of illuminated glass and fitted with blowers to lift the girls' skirts, startlingly yoking the strategies of girl show and fashion show.

The opulent nightclub that was most clearly the precedent for Ziegfeld's shows was part of New York City's Hippodrome, which opened in 1905 as an oversize consumption palace containing a gigantic theater, restaurant, café, and child entertainment center within one huge structure. The lush Hippodrome revues crossed the concepts of burlesque chorus line, circus, and masque, using wild animals, elaborate scenery, and what theater historian Robert Baral calls "armies of girls on view." [10] The themes of these spectacular shows—"A Trip to Japan," "Around the World," "A Yankee Circus on Mars"—headily celebrated a newly opened world poised for Americans as tourist and market sites, as well as locations of American expansionism enacted in the recent acquisitions of the Philippines, Puerto Rico, Cuba, and Guam.

Ziegfeld's stagings eventually equaled the extravagance of the Hippodrome shows, including such novelties as live circus animals and spouting fountains. The inclusion of a fleet of chorus girl/clothes models continued these related practices of ostentatious display and consumption. "Nothing is better than the hippodromic point of view in the glorifying of American young ladies," J. Brooks Atkinson commented of the later *Follies*.[11] The "hippodromic point of view" situated female spectacle within the larger spectacle of the world offered up as tour and colony. Because this worldview was also being sold in the era's department store displays, the Ziegfeld Girl linked political, commercial, and entertainment culture as the preferred showcase body.

Showgirls and the Ziegfeld Walk

Ziegfeld's mannequin/showgirl originated in his early ambition to highlight costuming in his shows for Anna Held. Held and Ziegfeld admired the elaborate dresses regularly used by their friend Lillian Russell in her performances, but Held was considered too small to wear that kind of costume. The implication here is that clothing must match a body, a "common sense" fashion dictum with specific social consequences, as the Ziegfeld enterprise illustrates. So Ziegfeld hired "twelve great big young women exactly of Lillian Russell's proportions," according to Held's daughter, "and when the show opened, these gorgeous girls walked on and off the stage as a background for the petite Anna Held. They neither sang nor danced—they were simply delightful to see. Thus the 'Show Girl' was born and thereafter Flo always used them in his shows." [12]

Ziegfeld interviews also allude to this beginning, and the showgirl became a hallmark of his theater style, as did the differentiations among women and body types. In popular theater of the time, the term "showgirl" was used interchangeably with "chorus girl" in most cases, although theater lore claims that producer George Lederer of New York's Casino Theater first made a distinction between "mere" chorus girls and the more "pulchritudinous" showgirls early in the century.[13] The Ziegfeld enterprise, however, brought this distinction into prominence, utilizing choreography that differentiated the dancers from the parading clothes model/showgirls. The costuming for all Ziegfeld Girls was costly and of high quality, but the showgirls in these productions were more directly connected with fashion modeling.

Ziegfeld revue costuming was renowned for being provocative but "artistic." For some of the showgirl spectacles, the staging and lighting, as well as the use of sheer fabrics such as chiffon, produced an illusion of nudity, when actually the women onstage were fully dressed in elaborate gowns. As a "special effect," this exemplifies the Ziegfeld enterprise in its split between the racy and the respectable, its conflation of costume and chorus girl, its identification of the body as high-priced commodity, and its management of sexuality through the values of consumer culture (chiffon evening gowns).

The *Follies* revues soon featured fashion displays as the focus of spectacle numbers. The signature Ziegfeld showgirl number was a variation on the fashion runway, an exhibition of outstanding evening gowns during a slow parade of beauties and musical accompaniment. This debuted with "A Palace of Beauty" in the 1912 *Follies,* in which showgirls were individually spotlighted as they crossed the stage one by one to the tune of "Beautiful, Beautiful Girl." The *New York Times* review of that show recognized that costume was being prioritized over chorus girl, describing the scene as "a gorgeous succession of effective costumes with girls who can carry them with good effect."[14]

The development of the clothes-model showgirl was furthered with the hiring of dance director Ned Wayburn for both the *Follies* and the *Frolics* in 1915, the same year that Lady Duff Gordon was hired for costumes. Traditionally, most revue chorus girls functioned as decor or background, simply twirling their parasols or swaying to music, with a smaller team of the more talented dancers brought forward for special

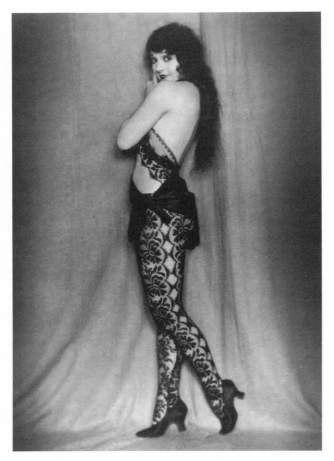

Mae Davis of the *Follies*, circa 1920. (Billy Rose Theatre Collection, New York Public Library for the Performing Arts)

numbers. In this traditional choreography, the dancers were divided by gender and degree of talent. Wayburn's innovation was to divide women by height, body proportions, and type of dance they could perform. The tall, clothes-model showgirls—the "A-team"—were used as a contrast in the *Follies'* huge spectacle numbers, in which the smaller chorines, the "ponies" or "chickens," performed dances entailing soft-shoe, acrobatics, tap, and bucks. The A-team paraded slowly down staircases or across the stage, exhibiting breathlessly elegant gowns, while the smallest women, the E-team, performed precision dancing in the mode of the British Tiller Girls, with the teams in between marked for the other styles of dance. "It was the anonymous 'ponies,' 'chickens' and 'A's' of the chorus that differentiated the Ziegfeld *Follies* from its rivals," as one theater historian explains.[15] The hype accompanying the *Follies* focused on the further differentiation of high-class fashion associated with this showgirl, emphasizing the hierarchical distinctions of both bodies and clothing.

Duff Gordon designed costumes for Ziegfeld from 1915 until 1921. The formal marriage of model and chorus girl occurred when Ziegfeld began to hire her models as well. " 'But they do not know how to sing or dance, let alone talk,' " the designer objected. "Ziegfeld assured her that all they would have to do would be to walk around and carry her beautiful costumes," Duff Gordon's biographer explains.[16] Her well-known mannequin Dolores (Kathleen Mary Rose Wilkinson) became one of Ziegfeld's stars, famous for her appearance in such *Follies* spectacles as "The Episode of Chiffon," in which she portrayed the Empress of Fashion.

At least one Follies Girl has attested to a backstage higher ranking of the showgirls over chorus girls, with Ziegfeld himself favoring the former. In public relations, Ziegfeld played both sides, defending the genuine talent of the dancers, denouncing the tall clothes model who could only walk and smile, but continuing to boast about the usage of avant-garde fashion. "The new 1915 model (Ziegfeld Girl) is not a show girl," the Ziegfeld persona claims in one interview. "She fills space of course, but she can also sing, dance, and talk." The next year, an essay supposedly authored by Ziegfeld touted the practical superiority of the chorus girl, claiming that the small, "agile" chorus girls make better wives than the tall, stately showgirls.[17]

Even after the departure of Duff Gordon, Ziegfeld shows continued to feature designer clothing. In two 1923 articles for the *Ladies Home Journal,* Ziegfeld explicitly describes his interest in avant-garde fashion. In the *Follies,* he claims in the first essay, "we not only influence but often lead the fashions. . . . If at times our clothes are exaggerated a bit and accentuated a little, it is because we must keep ahead." In the follow-up article, he explains that costuming might have to be replaced during the run of a single show "since these musical shows are dependent upon

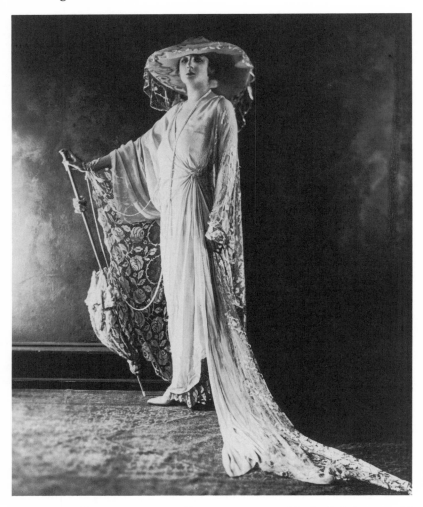

Dolores (Kathleen Mary Rose Wilkinson), epitome of the high-fashion model as Ziegfeld Girl. (Billy Rose Theatre Collection, New York Public Library for the Performing Arts)

and spread the fashions." [18] The practice of tying theatrical productions to merchandising was common before the turn of the century,[19] but its specific association with revue theater was Ziegfeld's distinction.

Another unique mark of Ziegfeld mise-en-scène was the costume that represented another commodity; the costumes "began to resemble objects rather than clothing," as one historian put it.[20] For more sensational effects, the women onstage were dressed as everything from taxicabs to soft drinks. Haute couture was often an important theme in these numbers, with the showgirl embodying high-fashion apparel items. This trend began with the 1910 *Follies* number "A Woman's Necessities," in which showgirls represented lingerie, corsets, jewels, furs, and other accessories. In the *Frolics* of 1919, they paraded as gems in the "Beautiful Jewels" number and as items in a bridal trousseau in "Laceland" in the 1922 *Follies*. The Ziegfeld Girl as this conflation of clothes *and* model was an influential early version of The Girl described by Ann K. Clark as "the abstract consumable and the abstract consumer," the ubiquitous, youthful media image which represents the exchange of self for commodity.[21] The Ziegfeld Girl is similarly abstracted, in spite of her individualized beauty and distinctive costumes, in this kind of exchange: "Beautiful Jewels," "A Woman's Necessities," time experienced as an episode of chiffon.

The haute couture fashion displayed in the *Follies* emerged at least partly as a way to represent exclusiveness and individuality, a response to the new mass-produced clothing industry at the turn of the century. At a moment when ready-made clothing served to democratize fashion, Ziegfeld's theater featured designer gowns made in Paris, London, Berlin, and New York, all of top-rate fabrics and hand-sewn trim. In the chorus girl economy, the Ziegfeld Girl had value precisely because this other market—the fashion industry, the culture of self-commodification—had so thoroughly permeated cultural concepts of identity and value.

The Ziegfeld Walk associated with these fashion images was specifically developed by Ned Wayburn in 1917 to parade the A-team showgirls. According to Baral, the Walk was "a combination of Irene Castle's flair for accenting the pelvis in her stance, the lifted shoulder, and a slow concentrated gait. A girl would enter into the spotlight very quietly—no smile visible. As she proceeded down stage, a small glimmer would appear, then, as she reached the center stage, she'd turn her full allure on to the audience." The parade downstage was usually a procession down a staircase. Unlike the traditional fashion walk down a ramp or runway, the Ziegfeld Walk was devised for a set of dramatically steep risers designed for Joseph Urban's *Follies* stages. Wayburn created a processional step suited to this architecture, which necessitated an unusually artificial thrust of hip and shoulder in order to keep one's balance.[22]

The Ziegfeld Walk is a logical element in the theatricalization of the fashion industry, a trend that was firmly in place with the popularity of the fashion show, a common urban merchandising technique by 1910. Yet the choreography of the Ziegfeld Walk and the replacement of the ramp with the staircase is also an organization of gender, with the regimented female body marched into laboriously artificial poses to accommodate an architecture. The choreographies of these numbers, which matched body types to movements and to costuming, exemplify the links between gender, commodities, and behavior. Moreover, as a discipline concerned with surveillance of self and others, this fashion choreography works across the axes of multiple cultural registers. The strained artifice of the Ziegfeld Walk can easily be read as the restraint and control of "the lady," an implicitly racialized image. Fashion analyst Jennifer Craik describes this more complex way that fashion as a social "instruction" articulates an identity: "Social and sexual identity," she writes, "is lodged in the way the body is worn. Gender—especially femininity—is worn through clothes."[23]

Female costume as an identity and self-knowledge was recognized by Ziegfeld himself, at least according to the Cantor and Freedman biography. Ziegfeld apparently insisted that the women's costumes be expensively lined: "He maintained that it was the quality of the lining against the bodies of the girls which made them act and feel more feminine, and enhanced their grace and movements on the stage."[24] Obviously there is a factor of male control here and a prurient imagination of women's bodies beneath the dresses. But to see this only as a kind of secret male voyeurism occludes the comprehension of "fashion" as a system of internal as well as external surveillance, a system in which consciousness is as important as visibility.

The behavior Ziegfeld required onstage, the "grace and movements" of specific social codes, is not something he invented or personally engineered. Clothes models, Craik suggests, act out a number of characteristics understood in Western culture as feminine: "the importance of appearance; fetishization of the body; manipulation and molding of the body; the discipline and labour associated with 'beauty' and body maintenance; the equation of youth with femininity; and feminine lifestyles."[25] High fashion alone would not have characterized Ziegfeld Girls without the coded body in a set of disciplined movements.

By the second decade of the century, Ziegfeld Girls would join cinema celebrities as voices behind endless newspaper and magazine articles giving beauty advice about diet, exercise, makeup, and skin care. Beauty routines were the offstage equivalent of the onstage choreography, particularly as the slimmer body became more fashionable over the decades. Two late-1920s publicity stunts of Ziegfeld Girls taking "pledges" illustrate the link between appearance and behavior. Photos of one event show the famous beauties signing the "pledge to slenderness," a document renouncing "the false pleasures of the table" because, as opposed to food, the supple figure was the truer "pleasure." In a related event, Ziegfeld Girls pledged the "Curves, Charm and Contour Club" whose members "will not be entrapped by long clinging skirts" or by "scanty, short ones." They will instead choose "moderately long and modestly short ones" enabling them to be "at the same time graceful and dignified." [26]

As this latter pledge suggests, the other offstage choreography famously required by Ziegfeld was "ladylike" appearance on the street. "A Ziegfeld Girl had to be a lady at all times," a former showgirl recalled. "She must do nothing to disgrace the name of Ziegfeld." [27] His longtime secretary Matilda Golden Stanton later confirmed that one of her jobs was to contact showgirls Ziegfeld had seen dressed badly on the street to tell them they "can't dress like that." In a 1975 interview for the *New York Times,* former Ziegfeld Girls remembered "how he insisted that his girls always wear hats, gloves, and high heels in public" and that he apparently managed details such as abortions for them as well. "Some girls must have gotten pregnant, but if they did, you never heard about it." [28] Comments like this appear so often in interviews and memoirs that we can assume that, even if not always practiced, the surveillance of private behavior was at least an element of the Ziegfeld backstage life.

This odd junction of privilege and proscription, surveillance and exhibition, suggests the contradictions of the fashion system itself. During the Ziegfeld era, 1907 to 1932, women's fashions changed dramatically, literally giving the female body more mobility and visibility with the end of corsetry and the appearance of legs and lighter material. On the one hand, fashion was a powerful apparatus in making possible the public woman who worked, shopped, and increasingly appeared in colleges and businesses. The avant-garde fashions of the Ziegfeld stage on some level addressed this more powerful, more independent female

consumer, those readers of the *Ladies Home Journal* who were being assured by Ziegfeld that the clothes in his productions were cutting-edge
style. On the other hand, the rigid on- and offstage choreography of the
showgirls resituates this more independent modern woman within decidedly restricted behaviors. The same fashions making women more
mobile during this era also made them more conscious of themselves as
measuring up to the expected "look." As one analyst more recently suggests, the meanings of fashion for women and its meanings in culture are
not necessarily the same. Fashion can be an apparatus of independence
and confidence, but women are also sociopolitical bodies, enmeshed in
power relations that fashion encapsulates.[29]

The three-dimensional tableaux of the A-team Ziegfeld Girls were directly related to department-store practices in the first three decades
of this century. Rachel Bowlby's elegant description of display-window
dynamics sums up the powerful mode of identification for the shop-
per/spectator. The glass window, she says, "reflects an idealized image
of the woman . . . who stands before it, in the form of the model she
could buy or become. . . . [T]he woman sees what she wants and what
she wants to be."[30] "What she wants to be" is a configuration of class,
gender, and race. The politics of this configuration are immediately foregrounded in the suntan injunction imposed by Ziegfeld on his Girls in
the 1920s. In the interview with former Ziegfeld Girls quoted above, the
women remembered an important detail of personal discipline: Ziegfeld paid the young women bonuses of two hundred dollars if they had
not become suntanned by the end of the summer.[31] Suntans had just become popular in the 1920s as class signs of leisure time and access to sea-
side resorts. The insistence on perfectly white, untanned Ziegfeld Girls
suggests the racial dimension of the showgirl-fashion model, although
other department store devices borrowed by the *Follies* had racial implications as well.

As fashion was more and more foregrounded in the *Follies,* the Ziegfeld Girl was described and publicized as a commodity item displayed in
a sumptuous setting. The 1915 newspaper article "Ziegfeld Trade-Mark
Asset to Chorus Girl" cited earlier in this chapter quotes Ziegfeld as the
honest shopkeeper claiming that people "have a right to get the worth
of their money. . . . They come to see the girls. There is nothing on

earth as beautiful as a beautiful girl. Isn't the most beautiful thing in the world worth putting into the right setting?" In other press releases, the shopkeeping metaphor is even more explicit: "There have been many descriptions of the 'Follies,' but I think none fits them more accurately than 'life's Show Window,'" the Ziegfeld persona proclaims, "for as we try to present them with the glorified girls, the galaxies of stars, and the marvelous scenic effects and costumes, we hold up to the world all the elaborateness and beauty that are to be associated with a shop-window of life."[32] The continuum between Ziegfeld's theater and the department store window was direct, in that the latter began to use more elaborate backgrounds and live models during this era. Macy's exhibited its spring fashions in 1914 as a Riviera promenade, for example, featuring beautifully costumed women strolling in a romantic setting.[33]

The emergence of the department store in the last part of the nineteenth century provided not only a respectable public place for women but also a radical democratization of consumership. Items were pre-priced so that bargaining was eliminated, and goods were displayed for customer perusal; no money was required to window-shop or browse. Yet despite this leveling of consumer access, the department store displays themselves linked consumption with class aspirations, appealing specifically to the upscale customer. Hence the themes around which stores were decorated suggest class interests and preoccupations. In 1903 New York's Siegel-Cooper store offered a six-week "Carnival of Nations" that included "Oriental Week," complete with Turkish harems and a "Cleopatra of the Nile." Imported commodities—the availability of which had sharply risen by the early 1890s—were made accessible within the fantasy of imported settings, so that a woman could purchase a Japanese shawl in a "Japanese garden," buying "not only the shawl but the exoticism injected into it," says historian William R. Leach. Fashion shows within the stores incorporated choreography and elaborate special effects in presentations such as "the Garden of Enchantment" and "Aladdin and the Wonderful Lamp."[34]

The department store offered the "experience" of the foreign and the exotic that could likewise be purchased by upscale consumers of the tourist industry, which had rapidly developed in the United States with the opening of the American office of Cook's Tours in 1873. Tourism as the confluence of spectatorship, consumerism, and exoticism was paralleled on the stages of this era's revues. Department store consumers purchased Japanese shawls in ersatz Japanese gardens and in the Ziegfeld revues consumed spectacles of "Oriental Love." For *Follies* theme numbers, American girls dressed up as Arabian, Burmese, or Siamese princesses and as "Turkish Bath Girls" in the vignette of this title, as señoritas in "In Sunny Spain," and as geishas in "Under a Japanese Moon." As Judith Williamson has said of contemporary "exotic" fashion, "the appropriation of other people's dress is fashionable provided it is perfectly clear that you are, in fact, different from whoever would normally wear such clothes."[35] Ziegfeld Girls exhibited themselves as daughters of the Nile or as maidens of Hawaii, but always with the effect of contrast: these are white American girls playing with costumes. Moreover, the difference enacted in revue exoticism was also the construction of sexual difference as exotic, priming the desirability of Ziegfeld Girls with the tease of double otherness: female body as sexually foreign but also as true Caucasian under the veils and turbans.

Commenting on this era's elaborate department store displays, Leach emphasizes the importance of the "concept of show" in capitalism's "culture of consumption . . . whether in the shape of a theatrical show, a baby show, a show girl, a showplace, or a showroom." He speculates that the desire to "show things off" worked as a resistance to more traditional American values of reserve, modesty, and thriftiness.[36] Female sexual spectacle operates with fascinating seamlessness in this continuum with baby show, showplace, and showroom. Paradoxically, although the Ziegfeld Girls' costumes were frequently provocative, the impact of the showgirl display was inevitably one of domesticization; like other glamorous commodities, these Girls were meant to be luxury items for the home.

Given the prior mythology of the chorus girl and her wealthy suitors, press releases consistently emphasized the Ziegfeld Girls as potential wives for well-to-do spectators. "Mr. Ziegfeld has difficulty keeping his beauties," a typical story ran, "because the millionaires so persistently carry off and marry them." Though even the most romanticizing theatrical histories admit that relatively few Ziegfeld Girls married into great wealth, the claim was often made in Ziegfeld press releases that "rich men, particularly rich men's sons, tend to look for and to find their heart's ideal in some beauty of the chorus." [37] Within the dynamics of the *Follies*, the chorus girl rich-marriage myth takes on further implications, not just guaranteeing the end of a career but also suggesting that, as the wealthy wife, the chorus girl continues her function as high-class decor. If this sounds like old-fashioned Veblen—the wife as ornament— perhaps this alerts us to the profoundly conservative nature of the Ziegfeld Girl as both a figure whose nudity is actually a chiffon gown and a figure of nostalgia for the Veblenesque moment when women were not part of public life.

Illusionists

The showgirl business was not the only Broadway entertainment "inventing women" with finery and elaborate accoutrements in the early part of this century. The Ziegfeld Girls in their headdresses and boas, with the lights turned down for special effects, look remarkably like another kind of fashion-performer popular during this time: men who made stage careers as "serious" cross-dressers. Male illusionists were a staple of American show business in the late nineteenth century and well into the twentieth. The best-known female imitator, Julian Eltinge, was still going strong in the late 1920s. In 1922, ads for the *Follies* ran alongside ads for Eltinge: "The Handsomest Woman on the Stage Is a Man."

Eltinge's most famous predecessor was Francis Leon, at the height of his popularity in the 1880s, who is often given credit as the founder of this particular impersonator tradition in the United States. His contemporary reviewers proclaimed Leon's performances were not burlesques of women but sincere, charming celebrations of femininity. The Only Leon, as he was called, insisted he did not use "costumes" but authentic women's apparel and accessories: petticoats, face powder, makeup, two-hundred-dollar gowns, and real lace undergarments. [38] The performances of Leon and his successors emphasized etiquette, grace, taste, and fashion, with the impersonators modeling the latest hair designs and gowns. Eltinge joined this tradition in 1905, proudly establishing a professional stage presence "always as a perfect lady," as a typical con-

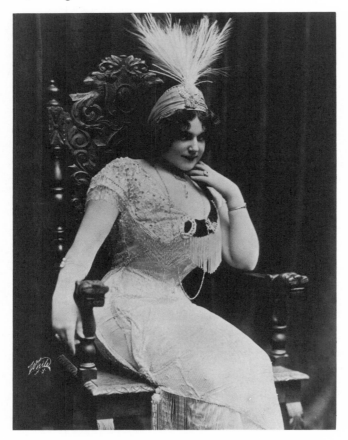

Julian Eltinge: "The Handsomest Woman on the Stage Is a
Man." (Billy Rose Theatre Collection, New York Public Library
for the Performing Arts)

temporary publicity article explains.[39] In 1907, when the first Ziegfeld
Follies featured a Gibson Girl scene, Eltinge was also using the Gibson
Girl as one of his roles.

Julian Eltinge won a wide and popular audience for the "magic" of
his transformation.[40] Nonetheless, Eltinge's reception was never entirely
positive. Along with rave reviews came nervous chiding about masculinity and normality—clearly a response to the visible gay male presence

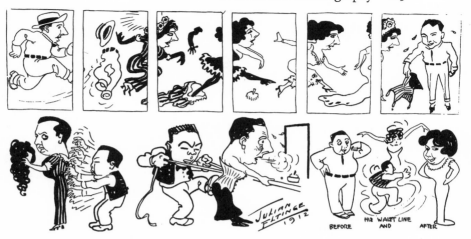

Newspaper cartoon commenting on Julian Eltinge, "before" and "after," 1912.

in New York City in the first decades of the century, when gay drag balls were also at the height of their popularity. Eltinge was forced to launch a never ceasing press campaign about his "real" masculinity offstage, his sports interests, and his ability to punch out threatening hoodlums at the stage door.[41] Obviously, questions of sexuality in relation to gender haunted his career: their alignments, their relationships, their permeability—and their relationship to performance and costume. A 1912 newspaper cartoon about Eltinge blatantly points out that the middle-aged man and the fashionable, wasp-waisted woman are separated only by corsetry.

There are striking similarities in these two projects: the Leon/Eltinge tradition of impersonation and the tradition of the Ziegfeld Girl. Both are performances of the "perfect lady," emphasizing authenticity, respectability, femininity, fashion, and—in the case of the *Follies'* nude effect—elaborate illusions about what was seen, suggested, and revealed. Ziegfeld's well-known obsession with costume detail—linings, buttons, fabric cuts—paralleled Leon's and Eltinge's discussions of these crucial elements of fashion and femininity.

Yet this very emphasis on costume and carefully choreographed performance exemplifies how easily that performance can be interrupted, turned inside out, with the subversive suggestion that sex and gender are *only* a matter of behavior and dress. The performances of Julian Eltinge openly revealed that gender as a costume need not bear any relation to the body and its desires. If, after all, the essence of "a perfect lady" is petticoats and face powder, then perfect ladyship is no more stable or reliable than that vanished ghost, the True Woman. Future drag queen artists would owe as much to Julian Eltinge as to the Ziegfeld Girl in her abundance of feathers and sequins, silks, and chiffons. In 1993, Howard Crabtree's production *Whoop-Dee-Doo!* at the Actors Playhouse in Manhattan acted out this inheritance with a drag queen version of a Ziegfeld-style revue show, starring nine men in glitz and headdresses.

At one point Ziegfeld aggressively advertised that he was looking for "natural" beauty and would not allow his showgirls to wear makeup onstage. But the Ziegfeld Girl's trademark remained opulence—the high-quality apparel and accessories, the veneer of feathers, sequins, and jewels. The excessiveness of costumes and special effects attests to the very nature of that sexuality as performance and imitation. Female imitators often appeared on the Ziegfeld stage in the vaudevillian portions of the program. These *Follies* "illusionists" performed, significantly, not in the refined tradition of Eltinge but in the more vulgar burlesque tradition. In the *Follies* of 1918, for example, comedian Bert Savoy played a huge, whorey redhead, foul-mouthed and tipsy—obviously *not* a Ziegfeld Girl. To bring the respectable Eltinge onto the *Follies* stage would perhaps have made too visible the props of the glorification project.

All this suggests that the priority of fashion in the *Follies* also worked in a sexual dynamic of projection and denial, part of the "guarantee" of female heterosexuality in the Ziegfeld Girl. If fashion works as a way to wear gender, with all its sociopolitical implications, it is a way to wear sexuality as well, especially in light of the importance attached to women's gendered clothing by the early sexologists. During this era in which female heterosexuality was tentatively being understood as less than inevitable, the stakes rose on the visual connections of gender and sexuality. This became the case especially as 1920s lesbians and feminists used masculine dress as deliberate marks of self-identification. In response, the very rhetoric of the New Woman and her questionable sexuality was co-opted into the language of commodification and advertising. Terms such as "independence," "self-fulfillment," and "individuality" gradually lost their feminist political impetus as they were redefined, through advertising, as possibilities latent in the choices of gown, hat, or cosmetics. Granted, feminist agendas in the early decades of the century were not directly related to recognitions of lesbianism. The point is that in co-opting feminist ideals as consumerist ideals, the economies of fashion worked to construct womanhood as irrevocably heterosexual, romanticizing the modern consumerist family and home.[42]

The changing understandings of female bodies in the first three decades of this century, with the attendant confusions of both sex and gender classifications, constitute what Marjorie Garber calls a "category crisis," an anxiety she attaches to the scene of cross-dressing. The popularity of Julian Eltinge attests to this anxiety in that his "magical" transformation opens the possibility that the categories of gender are themselves creations from trunks of clothes.[43] "Category crisis" perhaps also explains the *need* for cross-dressing acts on the Ziegfeld stage where, in the showgirl parades, the choreography of the feminine is so exactly proscribed in terms of accessories, behavior, class, age, and race.

And here we see the intersection of the Ziegfeld Girl's studied (heterosexual) respectability and her requisite whiteness. "Category crises," claims Garber, "can and do mark displacements from the axis of *class* as well as from *race* onto the axis of gender." What is acted out as crisis of gender may well be a manifestation of these other issues. Garber emphasizes in particular how racial and gender categories are crossed in politically efficient ways to control dominant interests. She gives as an example the practice of cross-dressing in minstrel shows, where Francis Leon made his start. As a result, "a black-impersonating female impersonator summed up and disempowered (or emasculated) two threatening forces at once." [44]

As the following chapter will detail, the category crisis of race was more visible in the United States in the first three decades of this century than was that of sexuality. However, the eugenicist argument for an "American race" — a "true" northern European Caucasian race as an American one — paralleled anxieties about a "true" female body. Not surprisingly, the Ziegfeld Girl, a sign of the "guaranteed" American female, often performed in café au lait blackface or in national or cultural drag—as Turkish harem girl, Japanese geisha, or Egyptian princess. These performances worked in the Ziegfeldian theatrical tension between the racy and the respectable, invoking a darker or Asian race but retaining the identity of the white girl beneath the costume.

CHAPTER FOUR

Racialized, Glorified American Girls

"Mr. Ziegfeld Says All These Girls Are Pretty"

The quotation above is the headline for photos accompanying an article signed by Florenz Ziegfeld Jr., "Picking Out Pretty Girls for the Stage," in a 1919 issue of *American Magazine*. The headline cites an authority but also suggests the posing of a real question that Mr. Ziegfeld has answered. In the photo captions, Madeleine Fairbanks is described as "straight American"; Lucille Levant "has blue eyes, blond hair, and, like other girls in these pictures, a short upper lip"; Gladys Loftus is praised for having "the unusual combination of dark brown hair and blue eyes, also of a straight, fine nose and a short upper lip." One young woman described as having a "slightly irregular nose" fortunately also has the saving "short upper lip," which presumably earns her the Ziegfeld nod.

"Picking Out Pretty Girls for the Stage" has been quoted frequently in recent scholarship because it includes a witty contrast of the Ziegfeld Girl's wholesomeness as opposed to the alluring vamp figure of the era—"The vampire is not a popular household pet."[1] The article's major question and topic, however, is what "types" could be considered "pretty girls for the stage." The obsession with the upper lip and the identification as "straight American" pinpoints the unspoken social question: not "What is a pretty girl?" but "Who can be an American?" "Straight Americans" have straight noses and short upper lips, as opposed to Jews, African Americans, and "mongrel" ethnicities suddenly populating northern American cities. Political cartoons during this time often pictured these undesirables as monkey-faced, with large, devouring lips. The more obvious political twist in the article "Picking Out Pretty Girls" is the assurance that these Ziegfeld-selected girls are "native Americans," in the parlance of the times: "not only are they native-born, but . . . their parents and grandparents and remoter ancestors were also natives of this country" (121). For 1919 readers, it would have been clear

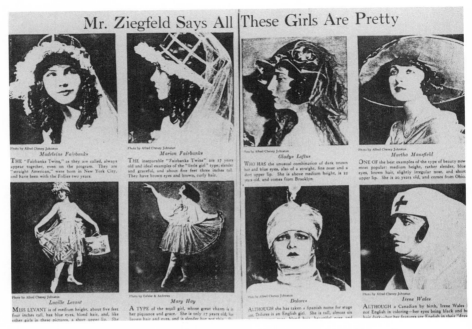

"Mr. Ziegfeld Says All These Girls Are Pretty." (*American Magazine*, December 1919)

that this meant not American Indian but "Nordic," which in the current eugenicist and nativist rhetoric meant the "American race."

In the first decades of this century, the Ziegfeld Girl was one of many sites where a national white race was being delineated along sexual lines. Other practices such as the beauty contest, the film and theatrical star industries, and magazine advertising similarly promoted Anglicized images of the American Girl at the exact moment when immigration from southern and eastern Europe, along with migration of African American populations from southern states, challenged nineteenth-century ideas of American identity. Ziegfeld's Glorified American Girl provides a particularly rich case study of this process because it left behind an extensive paper trail of publicity and an influential entertainment history, illustrating how a dominant image is circulated and how a "sexual plot structures [a] racial story," as Laura Doyle has written of the sex/race dynamic.[2]

Posing the question of the showgirls' origins, the Ziegfeld persona in a 1925 magazine article insisted on their geographical and ethnic diversity: "There seems to be no particular district or town upon which I can depend [for girls], just as there seems to be no one nationality or blend of nationalities that produces beauty. All nations, and all parts of the country, have the beauty potentialities."[3] These variations are supposedly illustrated in the accompanying photos of famous Ziegfeld Girls—Marion Davies, Mae Murray, Mary Eaton—whose individualized hairstyles and costumes signal differences solidly recontained within homogeneously Anglicized features and surnames.

Generally, the more democratic claims of Ziegfeld publicity ("You too can be a Ziegfeld Girl") contributed to grand erasures in the field of visibility through denials of difference or through the blind hope—no doubt shared on a large scale—that the melting pot would eventually serve up the face and coloring of Marion Davies.

The Glorified American Girl became the official Ziegfeld motto in 1922, but the identification of "American" Ziegfeld beauty began in press releases around 1914, during the pitch of anti-immigration politics nationwide. To examine how the Ziegfeld Girl functioned as a racial categorization, I explore three major strands of Ziegfeld's Glorified American Girl: first, the rhetoric of Ziegfeld's beauty-advice publicity, beginning in 1914, with its nativist and eugenicist overtones; second, the codevelopment of the Ziegfeld showgirl and the African American showgirl in the first two decades of the century, with the former identified as the "genuine" American Girl; and third, the construction of whiteness within the Ziegfeld shows, where the Glorified American Girl was defined as the contrast to racial and ethnic representations.

Certain Girls

Summing up his project in midcareer, Ziegfeld commented, "Women glorify gowns, and certain gowns can glorify certain girls."[4] As countless interviews and articles made clear, Ziegfeld was referring not only to the matching of girls with gowns but also to the particularity of "certain girls." The clothes required a body that presumably Ziegfeld alone could choose. While his dance directors often chose women for the tour shows, theater lore insists the only "real" Ziegfeld Girls were the ones selected by the producer himself. The selection of "certain girls" as Follies Girls was a major topic of Ziegfeld publicity that mystified and nationalized the audition process. A favorite theme of press releases and interviews, it is also the topic of three of the six national magazine articles appearing under Ziegfeld's name during the course of the *Follies:* "How I Pick Beauties," "How I Pick My Beauties," and the article quoted above, "Picking Out Pretty Girls for the Stage."[5] The latter emphasizes the great solemnity of the audition process: "Perhaps forty or fifty girls are tried out at a time. . . . There is no talking, no foolishness. . . . They are there for serious work" (126). This article also characterizes these potential Follies Girls as natural resources, native to this country: "There is not a section of the country that does not furnish its quota of pretty girls," the Ziegfeld persona claims. "No part of the country has a monopoly in this matter, but the South is one of the best sources of supply, and California is another" (34).

The industrial imagery of quota and supply appears in other news re-leases about the superior Ziegfeld product, with descriptions of young women lined up, inspected, and stamped (or not) for approval. News-paper stories emphasized the large crowds at auditions—"Picks 75 Chorus Girls from 3000 Aspirants," "Chorus Girls Swarm, 1000 Answer Call from Ziegfeld"—and feature stories played up Ziegfeld's selective eye: "When Is a Woman's Figure Beautiful? Florenz Ziegfeld Tells How He Judges."[6] The national reputation of the *Follies,* combined with the deluge of press releases on the selection and audition process, produced Ziegfeld as a prime national expert on female beauty, the wily indus-trialist on par with Henry Ford or Thomas Edison, processing national resources into glossy display items. In turn, the Ziegfeld office produced the persona of Ziegfeld the beauty adviser, whose "advice" was actually the definition of female beauty as racially white, nonethnic, and cate-gorized into "types" similar to those being used by the era's eugenics movement.

The Ziegfeld beauty-advice persona emerged from the publicity office in 1914, when the reputation of the Ziegfeld revue was solidly hooked to the Follies Girl. "The Ziegfeld trademark stands for beautiful women in daring costumes," an essay in the *Green Book* commented that year.[7] The beauty-advice column or feature story by then appeared regularly in popular media, supposedly authored by an actress or other female celebrity. As the sole selector of Broadway's elite bodies for show, the Ziegfeld persona was able to take on a similar expertise about women's hair, clothing, figures, and makeup. The premise and promise behind this advice was often, "You too could be a Ziegfeld Girl." A typical promotion, this one on behalf of a fan magazine's "personality contest," begins with Ziegfeld's announcement that it is "personality" that gets a girl into the *Follies* and encourages the female reader to "be jolly, happy, lighthearted." Just at that point of inclusiveness, the beauty expert then moves on to more exacting requirements: "I have said nothing about physique. Yet a beautiful rounded lovely figure is an attribute for the stage."[8]

Usually the Ziegfeld-voice beauty adviser was painstakingly specific in these press releases. Borrowing from popular discourses about the rules and measurements of beauty, typical Ziegfeld interviews describe "three distinct types" of beauty, "each with its own set of rules." In other articles, the Ziegfeld enterprise offers charts of these beauty types based on hair coloring—blond, red, or brunette, encouraging women to learn their types in order to select the correct hairstyles or clothes: "Florenz Ziegfeld Jr. Explains Why a Brunette Disposition and a Blonde Coiffure Are Sure to Make Trouble for Their Owner," one subheadline professes. Still other interviews specify measurements and ingredients: "These are the measurements that I consider about right for the girl of today. Height—five feet, five and a half inches. Weight—one hundred and twenty pounds. Foot size five." Accompanying this article, a chart of a silhouetted female figure illustrates the ideal dimensions and proportions.[9] The implication is that the Follies Girls' qualifications are the ideal for "the girl of today." Invariably, the specifications are exclusive, emphasizing the fine-tuned selections made by Ziegfeld, down to the size of shoe.

The charts, specifications, and measurements were common in beauty-advice discourses by the second decade of the century and were identical to the ones being plugged by countless other stars of the era. But their promotion as ideals of the Follies Girl offered not just a star to be admired or imitated but a nationalist identification as well. "How Pretty Is a *Follies* Girl? Evelyn Law of the *Ziegfeld Follies* Has Perfect Facial Measurements," one typical photographic feature proclaimed.[10] The category of identification, in turn, was reinforced by pseudoscientific language of other popular discourses describing physique, ethnicity, and race. Thus while these classifications and regulations of beauty, found in popular media from 1915 to 1930, are not unique to Ziegfeld's publicity, they provided evidence that a specific "American type" existed, as seen in the Ziegfeld Girl.

The language of specification and "types" fit easily into practices of Ziegfeld staging, as I described in the last chapter, where the smaller women or "ponies" were featured as the dancers, the medium-height women as "the backbone of the chorus," and the tallest women as the showgirls. In the language of many Ziegfeld press releases describing the shows and showgirls, the "types" of beauty are naturalized by a scientific order. "I measure the applicants who come to my office by the high types I have enumerated," the Ziegfeld persona declares in a 1914 news release. Feature stories about the Ziegfeld Girl selection often hyped the theater audition into no less than medical research. In one article, the Ziegfeld persona explains a scientific methodology for "determining the beauty of a girl's face. . . . For the facial test, I use a screen with figures marked on the frame. It is held before the applicant's face so that I can determine whether the eyebrows are level, the eyes on a level with each other, and the same distance from the middle line of the screen."[11]

The establishment of "types" was pervasive in the rhetoric of eugenics and nativism in the two decades before and after the turn of the century. The pseudoscience of physiognomy had been widely disseminated at the beginning of this era, with its appeals to a "naturally" superior Aryan "type" of head and features. While this particular offshoot of social Darwinism had declined by World War I, it was replaced by an interest in eugenics, a topic that permeated the popular press with editorials asking, "Is the Race Going Downhill?" and articles titled "The Rising Tide of Degeneracy: What Everybody Ought to Know about Eugenics." Eugenics as a science was closely allied to the politics of nativism, the movement to define a national race or a "true" American heritage that was Anglo-Saxon. This brew of racism and nationalism was evidenced in the revival of the Ku Klux Klan during this era and in a slew of supposedly scientific books such as Madison Grant's *The Passing of the Great Race* and Clinton Stoddard Burr's *America's Racial Heritage*, all of which deplored the "mongrelization" of America.[12]

The language of standardization and measurement, common in advertising at this time, had also become a tool of the eugenics movement, which sought to measure intelligence and character as racial character-istics. These tools of eugenics were utilized in the immigration debates; restrictionists recommended standardized tests to guarantee "quality" racial characteristics of potential immigrants. In this context, Ziegfeld's promotion of his "certain girls" as recognizable, standardized "types" resonated with specific nationalist and racial overtones. "I try to choose the American type," the Ziegfeld persona proclaims in "How I Pick Beauties." "There is a larger percentage of beauties in America than in any other country." [13]

During the period 1890–1920, the concept of Americanism was threat-ened less by foreign wars than by European immigration to this country. Indeed, American entry into the war heightened angry nationalist de-bates about the rising rates of immigration and the questionable loyalty of these new populations. Beginning in 1917, the rate of immigration nearly doubled over what it had been in the previous thirty years. More-over, whereas nineteenth-century immigration had largely originated in northern Europe, the latter waves of immigrants were increasingly from eastern European and Mediterranean countries. The two largest new populations were Italians and Jews, groups whose customs and cultural assumptions significantly differed from those of previous immi-grant generations.[14] Symbolizing the cultural threat from these groups and others, the new immigrants challenged the problem of what "an American" could be and what this American *looked* like.

The many attempts to create an American Girl in popular media during this era symptomized the need to impose a singular model (of Americanism, the American) against these confusing ethnic multiplici-ties and emerging concepts of what American modernity might mean.[15] Not surprisingly, local and national beauty contests became popular during this time as public judgments about the preferred best "look." A 1907 nationwide beauty contest sponsored by several newspapers, for example, selected Miss Margeurite Frey as first-prize winner for "her per-fect profile, her rose and cream skin, large, melting eyes, mass of crinkly, bright golden hair."[16] This model of blondness and fairness associated with northern Europe was eventually claimed by eugenicists as typical of the "American race," a rhetoric borrowed by the Ziegfeld enterprise for its Glorified American Girl.

The *American Magazine* article with which I began this chapter, in many ways a typical Ziegfeld beauty-advice text, strikingly illustrates how this discourse participated in the ongoing debates about immigration, nationality, and Americanism. A democratic pitch at first promises an open pluralism about beauty: "There are more types of pretty girls in America than in any other country in the world." The reason, we are told, is that "in the United States there are all the nationalities ever discovered; and that each one of them has its own special type of beauty" (34). But only one nationality is actually singled out for wholehearted approval in this piece. The Irish girl, it claims, is excellent " 'show' material" because she will usually have "nice eyes, a good nose, pretty hair, and an expressive mouth" (121). Martha Banta's comments on nativist thinking during this time period shed some light on this distinction. The prevailing popular hierarchy, she explains, included the Irish as being "at least imaginatively assimilable . . . these young Irish women were Northern European, Caucasian, and Christian, after all. . . . It was all the others—the Indians, Negroes, Mediterraneans, Asians, Slavs, and Jews—who could not be conceived of as being Americans." [17] The Ziegfeld persona concludes the "Picking Out Pretty Girls" essay with the proclamation about "native Americans" quoted above and reiterates that "there are more types of beauty . . . among strictly American girls" (121).

The nativist movement fashioned a racial underclass that was itself hierarchized, with African Americans at the bottom, followed by Eastern Europeans, Mediterraneans, and Jews, all of whom could be contrasted to top-tier "American" whiteness. Because the bottom tiers were collapsed into a single non-American category, the result was a binary racial structure that at least one anthropologist sees as analogous to gender categories.[18] The higher position of Jews within the non-American group could in fact explain a curious distinction made in "Picking Out Pretty Girls" about the presence of Jewish women among the "strictly American girls." "There are a great many very pretty girls among Jewish people," it assures us, "but they mature early and lose their youthful slenderness. For that reason they do not last long as chorus girls" (121).

This odd commendation/condemnation makes the presence of Jews within the Ziegfeld Girls deliberately ambiguous. (If they "do not last long," are they hired or not?) The tentative tone indicates an uncertainty about whether Jews can be considered Americans, the definition toward

which the article strains. Given the speculations about the Jewish identity of Anna Held, who died in 1918, the discussion of Jewish showgirls
may have been an oblique reference to the former Ziegfeld star. Held's
smallness and—especially in later years—her plumpness would have
disqualified her from the tall, fashion-model showgirl type promulgated
by the *Follies* after 1915. According to this article, her physical characteristics would only have reaffirmed a previous disqualification, because
the European Jew could not, of course, become the American Girl per-
sonified in the Follies Girl—at least not without a change of name and
identity (so that Marian Levy turned into Follies Girl Paulette Goddard).

The immigration debate in the United States was only one site of the
larger international eugenics movement spawned by various misapplica-
tions of Charles Darwin's discoveries and theses. By the second decade
of the century, the American popular press had disseminated it widely:
"Anything even remotely related to sex hygiene, infant mortality, birth
marks, baby culture, sex control, pre-natal influence, or to care, 'cure,'
or treatment of defectives is given a heading entitled 'Eugenics,' " one
scientist complained in 1913.[19]

Eugenicist research in the United States, girded by Darwinism and
supported by enormous endowments from Andrew Carnegie and other
private sources, gathered data supposedly showing that traits ranging
from criminality to nomadism to pauperism were inherited. Given such
scientific backing, American supporters of eugenics argued for steriliza-
tion of criminals and those who were "mentally unfit," but they also
argued blatantly against immigration, warning that "if we admit a single
immigrant of any race who is below the average of American intelligence, we have by that much lowered all the currents of American
life and character." Other arguments cited substantial differences in the
intelligence quotient (IQ) between "native and immigrant stock" and
made flagrantly racist cultural claims: "It is a great race alone that makes
a great poetry."[20]

The popular versions of eugenics may sound jingoistic, but the scientific versions were often as ideologically slanted. One paper at the 1921
International Congress of Eugenics argued that infant mortality among
poor immigrant groups should be seen as natural selection rather than
tragedy, a "natural" way of controlling an inferior population. Another

paper at the same congress concluded that the "Negro . . . is of right entitled to his freedom, to his opportunity, and to his pursuit of happiness; but he has no right to claim the exercise of these privileges at the cost of white man's civilization."[21] These arguments illustrate that the immigrant "problem" was grafted onto the larger racial problem and the growing resistance to the fact that Americans could no longer be described as white.

Madison Grant's *The Passing of the Great Race,* a wildly popular book that went through seventeen reprintings from its publication in 1916 to World War II, likewise exemplifies how the anti-immigration argument fused with African American racial arguments. This book also justified the necessity of selective infant mortality, dismissing "a sentimental belief in the sanctity of human life" and exhorting that "human life is valuable only when it is of use to the community or race."[22] Faced with the Caucasian categorization of most Europeans, including those deemed "undesirable" from Italy and eastern Europe, Grant cleverly posits three distinct "subspecies" in Europe to distinguish among supposedly white or Caucasion populations. The northern or Nordic race, from which the "American" race was produced, is physically and mentally the superior of the three. The stature of the Mediterranean subspecies is "stunted in comparison to that of the Nordic race and the musculature and bony framework weak" (18). The Alpine subspecies of central and eastern Europe produces a peasant type, but its worst representation is the Polish Jew, a "dwarf" type whom Grant imagines overwhelming the United States. The "true" American is "today being literally driven off the streets of New York City by the swarms of Polish Jews," he warns. Revealingly, the argument rapidly equates assimilation as sexual threat: "These immigrants adopt the language of the native American; they wear his clothes; they steal his name; and they are beginning to take his women" (81).

This invocation of seduction by an impure race suggests the close interaction of nationalist and sexual agendas. The women to be "taken" here are, by implication, young women of reproductive age. For eugenicists, this necessitated an urgent warning to racially pure white women about careful selection of breeding mates. The inclusion of "baby culture" and "prenatal influence" within the eugenics rubric made eugenics a woman's issue, often linked to patriotism. Grant minced no words about the need for women to be instructed about this, given female inclination toward recidivism: "Women in all human races, as the females among all mammals, tend to exhibit the older, more generalized and primitive traits of the race's past" (23).

Despite the eugenicist movement's contemptuous undertone toward women, a privileged, middle-class version of feminism was inevitably drawn to a scientific discourse that supposedly supported its goal of enlightenment for white women. The concern about immigration in relation to "sexual hygiene" is evident in feminist texts as early as 1895. A didactic New Woman novel of that year, otherwise devoted to the liberating activities of physical exercise, bicycling, and work for suffragism, warns forbiddingly of "immense foreign colonies in our midsts" and recommends that "strict immigration laws should be enacted and enforced to the letter. 'America for Americans' should be the watchword of all."[23] The sex hygiene instruction prevailed for more than twenty years. In a 1915 feminist book addressing "race responsibility," Florence Guertin Tuttle emphasizes the immense significance of choices by individual women about breeding: "To introduce into the precious strain of life undesirable citizens, in any way subnormal, is counter to the high purposes of each and an affront to so-called love."[24] The national issues here ("undesirable citizens") and the identification of clear scientific types ("in any way subnormal") are easily subsumed into the white woman's sphere and her presumed specialization of love.

Describing the deployment of the Western bourgeois body, Foucault emphasizes that eugenics would inevitably become a preoccupation for a middle class seeking its own well-being and continuation. Describing this "dynamic racism, a racism of expansion," he notes the high stakes involved for the bourgeoisie in its " 'cultivation' of its own body" because of what this body "could represent politically, economically, and historically for the present and the future."[25] The Ziegfeld Girl, publicized as "select" and true to American "types," was a high-profile site of such cultivation and nativist/eugenicist concerns. The very heterosexualization of this particular showgirl body—her association with feminine fashion, her mythologized fate into a wealthy (white) marriage, the "guaranteed" sexual authenticity of the Ziegfeld Girl—works in the same continuum as nativism's binary racial differences, demarcating an authentic body from its more threatening Others.

Ziegfeld Girls and Dusky Belles

The Ziegfeld "formula for beauty," as one reviewer put it poetically in 1917, was "a hip, a dimple, a skin as white as the moons the madmen see at morn."[26] Madness or, more specifically, white-black racial panic indeed characterized the perceived whiteness of the Ziegfeld choruses. Although the eugenics argument lumped together all nonnorthern European populations as nonwhite, blacks were specifically designated at the bottom of its evolutionary chart. Many scientists vigorously believed that African Americans were a separate species and even lower than southern European immigrants in their potential for assimilation; as one scientific publication claimed in 1916, "The Negro is fully as far removed from the white man as is the ass from the horse." Historian Kenneth R. Manning, who cites this ersatz analogy as an example, emphasizes in his work on race and science that during the era of eugenics, "being American and being black were antithetical concepts."[27]

Certainly in the United States at the time, African Americans were the most visibly marked nonwhite population. They were also legally bracketed into separate spaces; the 1896 "separate but equal" ruling kept Jim Crow laws enforceable in the North and the South alike. These "separate but equal" spaces operated in ironic and powerful ways in the New York entertainment scene, eventually establishing white and black musical revue traditions—Glorified American Girls in one, Creole beauties in the other—which visually undercut but ideologically strengthened the concept of absolute and biological categories of race.

Generally, the African American woman, especially the black chorus girl in her seductive versions of "high yellow" or "dusky belle," most definitively embodied the Otherness against which the Glorified American Girl had meaning. Within the Ziegfeld choruses, other non-Nordics could be bleached into American Girls (despite the fervent publicity swearing otherwise) by a change of name; Marianne Michalski was able to become Gilda Gray. But if any mixed-race African American women passing as white also passed the Ziegfeld chorus code, those scandalous secrets have yet to come forward. As I pointed out in Chapter 3, during the 1920s, when sunbathing had become fashionable, Ziegfeld paid his chorus girls bonuses at the end of summer for *not* getting suntans. As black Broadway and light-skinned black chorus girls came into prominence during that decade, the distinction of white Ziegfeld Girls became more urgent. Yet, paradoxically, the distinction was maintained not by exclusions of black performers and suntans but by specific appropriations of black entertainment and the representation of the dusky belle herself within the Ziegfeld shows, either named in songs or embodied in the light blackface makeup of café au lait described in the final section of this chapter.

The Ziegfeld enterprise is a complicated racial space precisely because of its interracial textures, layers, and backgrounds. Ziegfeld himself was undoubtedly a pioneer in racially integrated Broadway productions. His controversial move to feature black comedian Bert Williams as a principal in the *Follies* from 1910 to 1919 — the first African American to join a white cast — was richly rewarded by Williams's popularity.[28] Moreover, had Ziegfeld never produced a *Follies* revue, his reputation could have rested on his 1927 production of *Show Boat,* which virtually reinvented the American musical by breaking a number of racial and theatrical codes.

Unlike traditional musical comedies such as *Sally,* lighthearted excuses for song, dance, and chorus girls, *Show Boat* took on complex characterizations, tense subplots, and themes of miscegenation and racial conflict. Jerome Kern's music and Oscar Hammerstein II's libretto boldly reorganized the material from the 1926 Edna Ferber novel without euphemizing the social issues. In contrast to this frankness, for the 1929 film version the miscegenation theme was considered too volatile, especially for southern audiences, and was deleted. But instead of backing away from the racial issues, Ziegfeld broke from white theater tradition altogether by having the black Jubilee Chorus onstage at the same time as white players and at one point having them join a white chorus in counterpoint. Black actors played major roles, and Paul Robeson was the original and immediate choice for the part of Joe, singer of the perennially stirring "Ol' Man River." Robeson instead ended up in the later London version because the play took longer than expected to reach Broadway, but it was clear from the start that the first major musical to integrate its story and numbers would also be the first white musical to integrate its cast.[29] A number of African American songs and dances were included in the original *Show Boat,* and the black musician Will Vodery worked on the vocal arrangements for this and other Ziegfeld shows.[30]

The most haunting character in *Show Boat* is Julie, the biracial performer who passes for white and is married to a white man until the "racial truth" forces both of them from the troupe. The part catapulted white speakeasy singer Helen Morgan to fame, and she continued the role in the 1936 film version. Quickly recognizable as the tragic mulatto figure, self-sacrificing and doomed, Julie would also have been recognizable on 1927 Broadway as a "dusky belle," one of the many black female singers and dancers with Caucasian features and mixed blood, a figure of illicit desire usually associated with the "lowbrow" spaces of black musicals and Harlem nightclubs.

However, the dusky belle was not very neatly contained within those lowbrow spaces. Indeed, her growing prominence in theatrical entertainment since the turn of the century positions her not simply as the darker mirror image of the Ziegfeld Girl but more accurately as the origin and raison d'être of the latter figure. The circulated images of white women were dependent for their value on the presence and performance of other racial and ethnic identities. Beginning in the 1890s, the desirable African American female body "on show" in a parallel theatrical venue heightened the stakes of the upscale chorus girl's whiteness and in one sense necessitated the rhetoric of the Glorified American Girl. Overall, the two chorus girl categories illustrate how blacks and whites "invented one another," to use Henry Louis Gates Jr.'s elegant phrasing, how we "derived our identities from the ghostly projections of our alter egos."[31]

Chorus girls were an important feature in the all-black musical comedies and revues that played on or near Broadway between 1890 and 1910. *The Creole Show* (1890), *The Octoroons* (1895), *A Trip to Coontown* (1898), and *Clorindy* (1898) were the first black shows to succeed with white audiences, and their success enabled Bert Williams and George Walker's all-black hit *In Dahomey* (1903) to open in a major Broadway theater. Photographs from these black casts reveal that the male actors frequently used blackface to make themselves darker, minstrel-style, for comic effect, whereas the chorus girls were generally light-skinned or high yellow and often had Caucasian features.

The fascination of these young women for white audiences is evident in remarks by the *New York Times* reviewer of *In Dahomey* who was compelled to make a "minute inspection" of black bodies onstage: "The actors were dark, medium, and light," he reports. "Some of them were so light that they may have passed for white, except that the flare of a nostril, the weight of an eyelid, or the delicate fullness of a lip betrayed them to minute inspection. One of the chorus girls clearly had blonde hair that was not peroxide. She had a smile like the smile of Sarah the divine." [32] The urgency of his inspection is suggested by the small, fine details he can finally identify as African American — an eyelid, a nostril, a lip — as if, in his intense search for difference, he were standing at the footlights peering anxiously up at the stage. The search for difference and the simultaneous appeal of Otherness — the puzzle of the blond hair, the attractive "fullness of a lip," the Sarah Bernhardt smile — richly illustrates the cross-racial dynamic of desire and distancing, inclusion and exclusion, that fueled interest in the black revues and black chorus girls.

The light-skinned black women in the African American Broadway chorus suggest the predominance of white standards of beauty for women, as evidenced by the growing cosmetics industry, which pitched bleaching creams for whiter skin to white and black women alike. [33] These dusky belles also foregrounded the tensions and contradictions in the struggle for racial definition. Black chorus girls apparently offered to white audiences the thrill of a forbidden sexuality; the display of their light skin exposed miscegenation, cross-racial desire. On one level, "bad" white male desire is visually displaced by a "bad" — that is, colored — version of female sexuality. According to the eugenic beliefs of the time, miscegenation always "reverted" its product to the "lower" race, so that, as Madison Grant's popular book reported, "the cross between a white man and a negro is a negro." [34] Yet at the very moment when race was being postulated by the eugenicists as biological and irrevocable, black musical theater produced its attractive female chorus girls as bodies "suitable for show," with colors and features not those typically associated with blacks — blond hair that was not the result of peroxide, a smile that could have been Sarah Bernhardt's—and in some ways indistinguishable from the chorus girls of white revues.

White Broadway was ever attentive to the African American entertainment scene, sometimes hiring black songwriters, often simply appropriating black dances and songs or producing hybrids such as coon shouters. Ziegfeld was no exception. His earlier star Anna Held had successfully used the cakewalk dance and coon songs and had inaugurated the hit song "The Maiden with the Dreamy Eyes" by black songwriters Bob Cole and the Johnson Brothers. Ziegfeld was especially interested in the *Darktown Follies,* J. Leubrie Hill's all-black revue that ran from 1913 to 1916. In 1914 Ziegfeld bought some of Hill's acts for his own show and hired black performers to teach the choreography, though the acts were performed by his own white cast.

During that decade, the black musical scene drifted away from white audiences, establishing its successes and grooming its stars uptown. But in the 1920s, it returned to downtown Manhattan with a lively series of revue hits, so the racial identity of the chorus girl as "suitable for show" acquired even sharper significance. Generally, racial tensions had heightened nationwide after World War I, when hundreds of thousands of African American veterans returned to this country to find their places within it unchanged; over two hundred people were killed in race riots that broke out in twenty-six cities in 1919. Black migrations to northern urban centers increased after the war. Between 1910 and 1920, the black population of New York City increased by 66 percent. During those years, the area above 110th Street was rapidly transformed into what was called a black metropolis, a center of black population, culture, and entertainment. Other immigrant populations had brought their own theatrical traditions—most notably, Yiddish theater—but none posed the immense attractions of popular Harlem nightlife in the 1920s. Many of these nightspots were white-owned clubs with black performers, but in smaller clubs the audiences were often mixed. The police sought every possible reason to close down such "black-and-tan" places where "white persons intermingled and danced with blacks," as one New York judge described it in convicting a bar manager for operating a "dance hall" without a license.[35]

The 1921 hit that brought black theater back to white Manhattan was

Shuffle Along, an all-black musical-comedy romance by Eubie Blake and Noble Sissle. Its undisputed success inaugurated a series of revues such as *Dixie to Broadway* (1924) that shared the structure and performance styles of the white revues, including the ubiquitous chorus lines and at-tractive women stars such as Florence Mills. The overlap was so great that white critics occasionally complained that "pure African" entertain-ment or blackface humor was getting lost, resulting in "black performers in a white show." [36] The criticisms attest to the importance of racial defi-nition for this entertainment. In truth, the appropriations went both ways. The codependence of white and black Broadway revues, their constant allusions to each other, and borrowings from and imitations of each other exemplify what Ann Douglas has called the integrated nature of American popular culture, "if only by theft and parody." [37]

A publicity shot for *Dixie to Broadway* dramatically illustrates the cul-tural pressures of both differentiation and identification. The show ad-vertised "fifty Creole beauties," some of whom strike a leggy pose in this image, identical to chorus poses for Ziegfeld or the Shuberts, while a larger-than-life Aunt Jemima backdrop reminds us of their "real" iden-tity. The gargantuan Aunt Jemima overwhelms them, suggesting the preponderance of myth over body and fantasy over evidence. For white viewers, perhaps the looming mammy, maternal and nurturing in con-trast to the svelte chorus girls, was safer than the forbidden desirability of the sexy black bodies in the foreground. And for black and white viewers alike, the image sums up the two most prevalent stereotypes of African American women: Jemima and Jezebel.

The latter stereotype is rooted in the white fantasy that black sexu-ality is primitive, more exciting for its Otherness, a concept dating from slave days. Its embodiment in the Jezebel stereotype had been a comfort-able explanation of rape by white slave owners supposedly tricked and seduced by the "hypersexuality" of the woman slave. [38] The concept of black female hypersexuality was reinforced by medical and historical dis-courses of the late nineteenth century positing that the black race, as the lowest in the racial hierarchy, was marked by uncontrollable sexuality. Black women and prostitutes were identified with similar iconography in medical books as women with biological genital aberrations, clues to their degeneracy. [39]

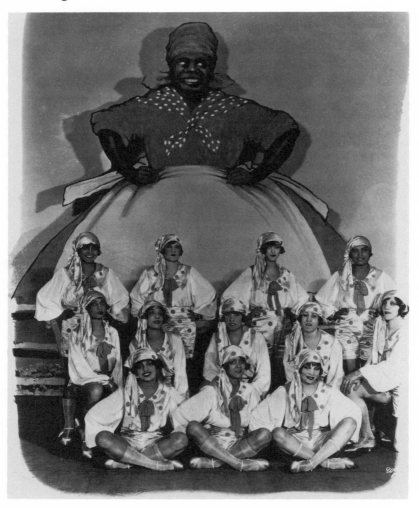

Chorus girls from *Dixie to Broadway*, 1924. (Billy Rose Theatre Collection, New York Public Library for the Performing Arts)

The Ziegfeld Girl as an upscale trademark was thus "guaranteed" to be absolutely apart from this different, seductive, but threatening parallel theater. Yet the white Ziegfeld Girl and the black chorus girl were similar not only in actual skin color in some cases but also in their cultural dynamics (as acceptable body on display) and visual dynamics (as leggy theatrical spectacle). So the definition of the white Glorified American Girl rested on the continual reestablishment of supposedly irrevocable boundary lines and demarcated racial spaces.

Generally, even if its players were ambiguously light-skinned, black Broadway maintained its blackness through its designation as a separate, lower cultural and social space. The labels of these white and black spaces as "highbrow" and "lowbrow" (at least within 1920s theater culture) are specifically racial in origin; for eugenicists, the skulls of "lower races" are closer in cranial shape to "the lowbrowed ape," whereas "the closer to western and northern Europe a people came, the higher their brows extended." [40]

These separate but unequal spaces created distinctions of class and aesthetics. As opposed to the relatively low-budget black revues, the more costly, extravagant white revues—most obviously, Ziegfeld's— were designated as the "real" Broadway. The high-class white revues were also considered "artistic"; in contrast, the appeal of black theater was ascribed to stereotypes about "natural" performance energy. Critic Gilbert Seldes in 1922 pronounced black Broadway theater as "without art, but with tremendous vitality." Admiring these shows, Seldes described their "appearance of unpremeditated violence which distinguishes them from the calculated and beautiful effects of Mr. Ziegfeld." The African American musical or revue, Seldes claimed, "is a continuous wild cry and an uninterrupted joyous rage . . . the élan vital is inexhaustible and unbridled and enormously good." [41] Seldes's enthusiastic ghettoization barely conceals his fear of black "unpremeditated violence" and "rage."

In 1921, Ziegfeld's musical Sally shared the kudos with Shuffle Along as the two top moneymakers on Broadway. Their story lines and production values sharply illustrate these differentiated spaces. Sally epitomized the backstage musical plot, the entertainment business's celebration of itself as the glamorous version of the American Dream. Its plotline sums up prevailing chorus girl mythology and specifically packages it as the upscale Ziegfeld trademark: the poor orphan Sally eventually becomes a star in the Ziegfeld Follies before her final-curtain grand wedding to a Long Island millionaire. Written as a vehicle for Marilyn Miller, the young dancer who had become the top-of-the-line Ziegfeld Girl in several previous *Follies, Sally* also featured well-known Follies Girls Gladys Loftus, Billie Dove, and, most strikingly, in her first speaking role, the mannequin Dolores, the former Lady Duff Gordon (Lucile) model, a reminder of the haute couture revue style.

In contrast, *Shuffle Along* is a political satire of behind-the-scenes election shenanigans in "colored" Jimtown. In good comedy fashion, the reform candidate, named in the enduring song "I'm Just Wild about Harry," triumphs by winning the mayor's office and the girl (later played by Florence Mills). The reviews of *Shuffle Along* often pointed out the "crudities of production" even as they praised the exuberance of the dancing and comedy, including the comic antics of the end-of-line chorus girl, newcomer Josephine Baker. Vaudeville-style comedy and energetic black dance numbers—the shimmy, the buck-and-wing, the Texas Tommy—characterized the show as much as the grand production numbers characterized *Sally*.

Both shows encapsulated elements the American musical would absorb and duplicate for decades, especially in cinema. As moving pictures took over the American musical, black musical elements would be whitened beyond recognition as they were relocated into more glamorous (white) trajectories and productions. Ziegfeld-style opulence and black music were often spliced together as in the "I'm Just Wild about Harry" number sung by Judy Garland and revisioned in the byzantine choreography of Busby Berkeley for the film version of *Babes in Arms* (1939). For the most part, backstage film musicals (musicals about show business) kept their African American inheritance not just backstage but offscreen, or they acknowledged it through blackface minstrelsy by Al Jolson, Eddie Cantor, Judy Garland, Mickey Rooney, and others, which in effect displaced black performers. Josephine Baker took her funny, eccentric, very sensual showgirl persona to France and to French films rather than American ones.

On Broadway in 1922, the two chorus girl traditions, black and white, made straightforward acknowledgments of each as the meaning of the other. That was the year the Ziegfeld enterprise began its glorification campaign, immediately imitated by the all-black revue *Strut Miss Lizzie*, which promoted itself as "Glorifying the Creole Beauty." The same year, the *Ziegfeld Follies* included a song about the growing visibility of black entertainment, "It's Getting Dark on Old Broadway," conceding that the Great White Way was no longer so, given all the "pretty choc'late babies" dancing on Broadway's stages and streets.[42] The song title's allusion to the lights of Broadway and the pun on "getting dark" startlingly names Broadway as a racial space rather than a neon space, the famous glittery lights of the White Way upstaged by a more surprising black-white contrast.

The staging of this number in the 1922 *Follies* imaginatively enacted the acknowledgments and anxieties of cross-racial desire. A lighting effect caused the chorus girls and their white costumes to take on a brown tint as they danced, so they were instantly transformed into dusky belles. As the song ended, the lighting picked out their white dresses and made their bodies "recede into undistinguishable black," according to reviewer Seldes. The total effect was whiteness to brownness to predominance of (white) costume over body. The image sums up the ghostly projection of beautiful, black, "primitive" bodies, used to fetishize the blondness and fashionability of the Ziegfeld enterprise. The substitution of white for black bodies also enacts the wider appropriation of African American musical traditions — Ziegfeld's purchase of acts from the *Darktown Follies* and his usage of African American choreographers to instruct white dancers. At the conclusion of the number, Seldes reports, the voice of singer Gilda Gray rose "in a deep and shuddering ecstasy" to the cry that ended the song: "Getting darker!" [43]

The "ecstasy" may well have been both Seldes's and the singer's, but the latter's thrill of cross-racial identification reminds us that white racial fantasy is not exclusively male. The mythology of black hypersexuality, a fantasy again buttressed by "closer-to-nature" primitivism, is fueled by white female fascination as much as white male anxiety. Besides, the black theater/white theater tensions were enacted as much through discourses such as fashion as through discourses about miscegenation. Ziegfeld Girls could safely "recede into undistinguishable black" because the spotlight would eventually return them to their positions as haute couture bodies. The very designation of the fashionable "lady" as a white woman ensured that black Broadway would always be kept in its place as far less posh, less elegant, and less socially valuable than the white revue tradition.

The *Ziegfeld Follies* and *Darktown Follies* required each other. But the latter also necessitated the urgency of the Ziegfeld show's nationalistic rhetoric, the declaration that it could indeed designate a "real" America and "real" American entertainment via youthful female sexuality in an age when "being American and being black were antithetical concepts." By 1925, the advertising logo for the *Follies* was "Florenz Ziegfeld Glorifying the American Girl, an American Revue Made in America for Americans."

Black and Tan

The black-and-tan cabarets of Harlem were perhaps the most transgressive sites of interracial flirtation in the New York theater scene during the latter years of the Ziegfeld era. Despite the publicized "strictly American" whiteness of the Ziegfeld Girl, however, the larger Ziegfeld revue stage functioned from the start as a more distanced kind of black-and-tan entertainment by including hybrid performances such as coon songs, blackface, explicit black comedy featuring Bert Williams, and the alluring "feminine" or high-yellow blackface, café au lait.

Eric Lott has argued that "the racial unconscious" is per se a hybrid scene of mixed desire and anxiety. The grotesqueries of blackface, says Lott, are not simply white projections of disgust so much as recognition of common identities.[44] The fear and fantasy is that racial boundary is by no means absolute. The decades-long obsession to enact blackface is an eroticized fantasy as well, a mixture of pleasure and threat. Given this landscape of mixed fear and desire, the visual dynamics of early black musical comedy make sense: black men in grotesque blackface and black women who comply to white standards of beauty economically sum up for white audiences the transgressive thrills of the white racial imagination. The fascinated 1903 reviewer of *In Dahomey* discovers, in his "minute inspection" of the bodies onstage, his own desire: "the delicate fullness of a lip."

Lott's focus is nineteenth-century minstrelsy, especially the blackface minstrel show, which he describes as literally "the first, formal public acknowledgment by whites of black culture." [45] Blackface performance was still alive and well in the first decades of this century, certainly in the world of the Broadway revue. White female singers and comedians often used this device to cite and sensationalize black sexuality. Blackface comedian Maude Raymond was famous for her line, "Golly, I'se so wicked," and Trixie Friganza's best-known song was "I'm Glad I'm Married," sung with Anna Held's coy gestures and knowing smile. Cecil Spooner was known as a "dainty, effervescent and charming bit of femininity" — certainly an Anna Held "type" — and was one of the most acclaimed blackface performers.[46]

While Ziegfeld Girls were discouraged from getting suntans, their stage appearance sometimes included the feminine version of blackface, "ginger" coloring or café au lait, the light-brown cast simulated in the sepia lighting effect of "It's Getting Dark." This skin color signified "naughty" sexuality; "I'm full of spice, sporty but nice," as one song put it, "sport" being slang for lovemaking. The song was "Miss Ginger of Jamaica," a number in the *Follies* of 1907 featuring Grace LaRue singing of her charms as "an elegant importation" known for "doing things up brown." [47]

Ziegfeld Girls in café au lait makeup are perhaps the apotheosis of the circular logic of blackface: representing "bad" sexuality, they also remarkably imitated the light-skinned black chorus girl from the competing theatrical tradition, who was in turn the "bad" version of the white chorus girl. As theater historian Rosaline Stone put it, these performances enabled Ziegfeld Girls to maintain that "white women were 'purer' since they did not behave in such a sexually permissive manner, but a 'woman of color' could supply sexual adventure and satisfaction." [48] The Ziegfeld Girl's imitation was permissible precisely because it was identifiable as disguise. Beneath the café au lait makeup was the American Girl who could safely act out the (bad) sexuality Ziegfeld Girls supposedly did not have. Nevertheless, for the Ziegfeld Girl to conjure up the black chorus girl was to acknowledge her, not as object to be imitated but as source and ground of identification.

A related, racially hybrid performance seen in the *Follies* was coon shouting. As my previous discussion of Anna Held pointed out, Jewish women such as Fanny Brice and Sophie Tucker are particularly interesting examples of this practice, which further complicates the black-and-tan fantasy by intermingling two marginal groups and traditions.[49] A beloved nugget of theater lore, repeated in films and biographies, is the first meeting of Fanny Brice and Florenz Ziegfeld: his admiration for her burlesque performance and his immediate contract offer that launched her from the Lower East Side to the *Ziegfeld Follies*. But what attracted Ziegfeld to Brice's performance was perhaps this double allusion to two cultures "when he heard Fanny sing 'Sadie Salome' with a Yiddish accent in a Broadway burlesque," as one description has it.[50] "Sadie Salome" is a coon song, as was the song Fanny Brice performed in black dialect for her 1910 *Follies* debut, "Lovey Joe."

Sophie Tucker, whose association with the *Follies* was brief, also used this hybrid style. Early in Tucker's career, she appeared in high-yellow blackface as "Sophie Tucker, the Ginger Girl, Refined Coon Singer." In her autobiography, Tucker claims she was considered too "big and ugly" to be taken seriously on the stage, so blackface was an acceptable comic mask. The dresser blacked her up, tied a red bandanna on her head, and with lipstick painted her "a grotesque grinning mouth." No doubt the mask also sanctioned an outlaw sexuality, the raucous physical yearning expressed in many of her songs. Her coon shouting in the *Follies* of 1909, sans blackface, won her such wild audience acclaim that star Nora Bayes jealously had her dismissed from the show.[51] For Bayes, Tucker's performance may have cut too close to her own specialization, which included not just her well-known "Shine On Harvest Moon" but "Oh You Beautiful Coon." Unlike Tucker, Bayes—the former Leonora Goldberg of Cleveland—repressed her Jewish identity, as did many Jewish performers.[52]

Many of the coon songs performed in the *Follies* referred directly to "dusky belles," such as the Queenie figure in the 1907 song "Handle Me with Care." A "dusky little maid" is celebrated in "Come Down Salomy Jane" and in "Miss Ginger of Jamaica." "Strut Miss Lizzie," borrowed from the 1922 black revue of the same name, describes "dusky belles" dancing and prancing with their beaux. As "specialty acts," these performances of minstrelsy, coon songs, and ethnic humor seamlessly appropriated what were then unquestioned mainstream entertainments. Comedy routines lampooning Irish, Italian, German, Jewish, and African American identities, reinforcing blatant stereotypes, "were considered hilarious and appropriate entertainment from approximately 1880 to 1920," as Fanny Brice biographer Barbara W. Grossman reports.[53] In a remarkable 1910 interview, black comedian Bert Williams suggested that theater caricatures are coping devices, cautious ways of allowing new, strange identities to appear.[54] Williams himself often performed in an exaggerated clown blackface, a mask of grotesque comedy acceptable to white audiences as the performance of blackness.

While there was wild enthusiasm and acclaim for Bert Williams and Jewish comedian Fanny Brice, as *Follies* stars they were situated in the ambiguous intersection of stardom and social contempt. Williams's elegant image in a tuxedo appeared on the covers of sheet music, but he was not entirely welcome by some white stars backstage, and when the *Follies* shows were on the road, he used the back elevators at hotels. The first, undocumented biography of Williams claims that the black performer himself insisted on the famous clause in his contract forbidding him from appearing on stage at the same time as the Ziegfeld Girls. This was supposedly done for his own self-protection; in return, Ziegfeld promised not to take the show to southern states while on tour. But Williams's later biographer, Eric Ledell Smith, finds no such evidence of Williams's intentions. Given Ziegfeld's usual tactics and the amount of press attention to the Williams contract, critic Gerald Mast suggests that the no-girls-onstage clause may have been another Ziegfeld publicity stunt.[55]

Likewise, Fanny Brice may have equaled any of Ziegfeld's female stars in salary and fame, but the wider social milieu and the *Follies* themselves categorized her otherwise, as a contrast to the Glorified American Girls. As Grossman points out, "Brice did not conform to the prevailing notion of female beauty and, more specifically, to the Ziegfeldian definition of it. . . . Whereas in burlesque she looked fine because there were so many sizes and shapes around her, Ziegfeld's elevated and homogenized standard of beauty exaggerated her difference from the norm." She was, as another biographer put it, "a natural contrast for the far-famed *Follies* Beauties."[56] Brice's initial appearance playing herself in the 1936 film *The Great Ziegfeld* illustrates this fairly dramatically. Two scenes after a major production number featuring cookie-cutter *Follies* showgirls, Brice appears onstage in a burlesque house introducing what she calls "gorgeous girls" of varying weights and heights, obviously coded as comically unattractive. Brice's physical difference from Ziegfeld Girls served her comic genius well, although in 1923, she buckled under to cultural standards and had plastic surgery on her nose.

The point here is that Ziegfeld's revue, far from being entirely white, created a more complicated space of various hybridizations, inclusions, and exclusions. Certainly the most exclusive space, and the one that received most constant press coverage, was the tableaux spectacles of the Girls, elegantly costumed and coded as class value—but also as racial/national value. The *Ziegfeld Follies* achieved the reputation of "the *Rue de la Paix* of American Femininity," as a fan magazine put it, and certainly not for the ethnic/racial comedy routines.[57]

Edmund Wilson realized some of these racial implications in 1925 as he watched a *Ziegfeld Follies* rehearsal and later wrote a short, impressionistic piece on what he observed, including "the negro wardrobe woman" whom he sees waiting backstage, "patient and with a shade of sullenness." Reading her "sullenness," Wilson begins a commentary alluding to the exclusion of blackness not only in this particular display but also in the aesthetic standards making the display possible. More specifically, the acknowledgment of the black woman as background moves Wilson to comment on the whiteness of the performers. Any ethnic differences among the performers themselves are absorbed into this definition as nonblack and therefore of value. As for the black female onlooker herself, she too is absorbed, through Wilson's prose, into a masculinized ("handsome") and invisible spectatorship, finally displaced altogether by the spectacle:

Behind [the Ziegfeld Girls], the negro wardrobe woman waits, patient and with a shade of sullenness—knowing herself handsome in another kind, she bides blinking at all that white beauty—those open-eyed confident white girls in their paradise of bright dress: turquoise skirts and canary-yellow cloaks, pink bodies hung with dark green leaves, white flower-stalks blooming into hats of purple and orange—all excited by the costumes and the music, proud to have been picked out by Ziegfeld, happy to look like magazine covers—brown-eyed, clear-skinned, straight-backed, straight-browed.[58]

The whiteness produced by Wilson's description duplicates the whiteness produced by the Ziegfeld enterprise through its constant need to distinguish, to define, and to allude to the Otherness by which an

American Girl can be determined. Ironically, Wilson's article includes, in an earlier section, a description of the costume colors and patterning of the choreography that enacts this defining of difference: "The show girls—white, green, white, white, black, orange; purple, green, orange, black, white, green. 'You've got two white ones together! Put somebody between them. You go over on the end, Gladys. Now, begin again!' " [59] Unwittingly defining whiteness in his essay, Wilson has in fact "put somebody between" the reader and the showgirls, someone who can silhouette, from behind, the "pink bodies."

CHAPTER FIVE

The Ziegfeld Girl and Hollywood Cinema

A 1925 Ziegfeld press release boasted that "one glance at the newspapers and magazines will show instantly that '*Follies* beauty' is a standardized term used clearly to convey a meaning that the entire public understands."[1] My argument in this book has been both an amplification and a complication of this claim about trademarking, public representation, and standardization. By 1925 the Ziegfeld showgirl had certainly become a cultural icon, whose recognizable image and meanings ranged from "strictly American" to haute couture fashion and household pet. Likewise, the stardom of Ziegfeld himself, his quasi-mythical stature as a Broadway "character" and creator of women, had been well established by that date. Together, Ziegfeld and his "Follies beauty" made up a glamorous legend that was enticingly open ended, featuring a powerful Pygmalion and an ever unique but renewable Girl.

Given this widespread cultural recognition, the Ziegfeld showgirl legend was destined for Hollywood, which—with the advent of sound cinema in 1927—would both immortalize her and displace her. During the next six years, revue-style spectacle was adapted to film musicals just as the great revue tradition of Ziegfeld, Earl Carroll, George White, and the Shuberts was sinking into its sunset on Broadway. Despite the bravado of the Ziegfeld news release quoted above, his *Follies* by the late 1920s "were coming to be perceived as lumbering dinosaurs," as one historian of the revue show points out.[2] Yet the film musical venue that deposed the brand-name revue Girl would in the long run glorify her as exuberantly as the original Ziegfeld shows, ensuring her presence in popular culture for decades.

As Gerald Mast has put it, "In the eyes of Hollywood . . . Ziegfeld came as close as any showman ever did to God Almighty."[3] And no wonder. The Ziegfeld enterprise offered narratives, character types, and visual styles highly compatible with mainstream Hollywood film: a showgirl with a Cinderella story line ("Discovered by Ziegfeld!"), a glamorous mise-en-scéne, excessive spectacle of every kind, and a heterosexual, up-scale closure (marriage to the millionaire in the front row). The Ziegfeld Girl was fated to be enacted by the likes of Lana Turner, and Ziegfeld himself proved irresistible for Hollywood representation as the godlike entrepreneur who could create and "glorify" women. For at least two generations of film audiences, from the 1920s through the 1940s, the Ziegfeld history offered a rich archive of shared cultural knowledge and assumptions about female spectacle, not necessarily connected to female talent but always associated with extravagant and opulent staging.

For later generations, Hollywood cinema remained the major source of knowledge about Ziegfeld and the Ziegfeld Girl, especially as 1930s and 1940s musicals began to be recycled in the 1960s through the main-streaming and influence of camp. Camp culture has both reread and endeared to us the excesses of these films, especially the grand pro-duction numbers that imitated those of 1920s Broadway revues. While these films easily lend themselves to the ironic interpretations of camp, they also provide rich historical readings for scholars and film lovers. The uniqueness of the musical as a genre, the proliferation of this genre through the depression and the war years, and the appeal of its stars—Ginger Rogers, Ruby Keeler, Joan Blondell—have directed a good deal of critical attention to many musical films with particularly Ziegfeld-esque markings.

Film history and camp culture have most lastingly delivered Zieg-feld's style and showgirl through choreographer/director Busby Berke-ley, who worked as an apprentice to Ziegfeld late in the latter's career and who has frequently been cited as the heir or "son" of the famous showman of pageantry. Film scholars and cinema buffs alike are familiar with Berkeley's excessive female spectacles, in which the camera tracks aggressively through the spread legs of hundreds of chorus girls. Berke-ley's chorus girls have been described as abstractions or as witty literal-izations of women as plastic images, "the image of woman as image," as Lucy Fischer puts it.[4] In production numbers that create imaginative, impossible spaces outside the narrative, the chorus girls are often liter-ally transformed into physical objects—gold coins, powder puffs, cans, violins—in the signature Ziegfeldian tradition of the melded costume and female body.

Indeed, the Berkeley aesthetic is a perfect cinematic match for Ziegfeldian aestheticizations and fetishizations. Berkeley's choreography and grand production numbers in films such as *Footlight Parade* (Lloyd Bacon, 1933) and *Dames* (Ray Enright, 1934) are often acknowledged as tributes to the elaborate dance and pageant numbers in the *Follies* revues: staircases, showgirls, visual gimmicks, and an abundance of feathers.[5] The relationships between pre-1930s musical theater and the development of the Hollywood musical are vividly foregrounded in these films. Berkeley's work illustrates what Martin Rubin has termed the "tradition of spectacle," the "showstopping" moments that work against or outside of coherent narrative.[6] The chorus girl spectacle of film musicals—the cookie-cutter line of leggy chorines—was a standard showstopper element directly inherited from the musical theater influenced by Ziegfeld.

The combined influence of camp, nostalgia, musical-genre history, and auteurist interest in Berkeley have canonized many of the major cinematic tributes to Ziegfeld, which are often quoted as key moments in cinema history or kitsch. Late-night television audiences might not sit through all three hours of the 1936 biographical film *The Great Ziegfeld,* but they may have seen its over-the-top showgirl spectacle "A Pretty Girl Is Like a Melody," re-created by Busby Berkeley in the 1941 *Ziegfeld Girl.* They may also have seen this number quoted in *That's Entertainment* (Jack Haley, 1974), the MGM self-promotion piece that featured this Ziegfeldian display as the ultimate grand production number.

As this suggests, cinema has provided for later generations glimpses, if not reproductions, of the lost world of Ziegfeldian revue. The *Follies'* showgirl tableau—part masque, part parade, part fashion show—has largely disappeared from theater culture. However, video stores carry or can order the showgirl film coproduced by Ziegfeld himself, *Glorifying the American Girl* (Millard Webb and John Harkrider, 1929), which climaxes with some stunning production numbers of women fantastically costumed as butterflies and cocoons, posed in equally ornate settings. A *Follies* butterfly-theme grand production number is also staged for the finale of *Sally* (John Francis Dillon, 1929), the film adaptation of Ziegfeld's stage hit. Enactments of Ziegfeldian numbers can be seen as well in *Ziegfeld Girl* and in Vincente Minnelli's *Ziegfeld Follies* (1946), which attempted to re-create an entire Ziegfeld revue.

As a site of titillating female images, cinema had always paralleled the world of revue theater. Between the debut of Anna Held in 1896 and Ziegfeld's first *Follies* revue in 1907, filmed or "canned" versions of female spectacle were already becoming commonplace. In one-reeler films seen at the nickelodeon, in the arcade, and in vaudeville shows, a woman's ankle or knee might be revealed by mischievous winds or a cheeky shoe clerk. The all male audiences of "smoking concert" films could glimpse even more—petticoats, garters, or suggestive voyeuristic scenarios.[7] These early, comparatively lower-class entertainments were so clearly nonthreatening to the revue scene that Ziegfeld included a sample of this new technology in his 1907 *Follies*. In a novelty skit, a motion picture portrayed Anna Held's face as the face of a comet zooming across the sky, a special-effects background for an onstage song. Emphasizing the status of the "canned" Anna Held as no more than a newfangled trick, Ziegfeld publicity boasted Held's refusal that year of a five-thousand-dollar moving-picture company contract. Subsequently, a few *Follies* numbers used film footage for special effects or to satirize cinema as a competing, inferior form. For a 1915 skit, "Commotion Picture," Ed Wynn imitated D. W. Griffith and provided live narration while a comic film was projected on a screen, showing a disastrous attempt to film the *Follies*. The next year, Ann Pennington debuted onstage via a film segment in which she was madly running, "Escaping the Movies," until she stepped from behind the screen to appear in person.

By the 1920s, cinema was not as easily reduced to a funny gag, and "escaping the movies" became a more serious preoccupation for Ziegfeld. The tableau spectacle, on which Ziegfeld lavished so much money and loving attention, was now in competition with the more fascinating visual phenomenon of motion picture editing, the picture that not only moved but could also jump from location to location, view to view, untethered from even the best front-row seat of a theater. Moreover, the camera enabled what no privileged theater seat could possibly provide: the close-up of the dimpled knee. Certainly the technologies of the close-up and shot-countershot were vehicles for the further fetishization of the showgirl figure from theater lore.

Silent movies with chorus girl heroines, such as *A Chorus Girl's Romance* (1923) and *The Great White Way* (1924), had been popular before the advent of sound technology in cinema, but the development of

such technology made it possible to deliver an entire Broadway musical on screen. As one newspaper report excitedly described it, "patrons
of every crossroad village movie house" can "see and hear high-priced
Broadway performers."[8] In 1929, tickets to Broadway productions aver-
aged $3.00, with the best seats $6.50—the equivalent of about $130 today.
Tickets to the movies cost thirty cents or less. Mass audiences who
could not have afforded tickets to Ziegfeld's Broadway shows and tour
shows were promised "honest-to-Ziegfeld songs and dances" in ads for
Mervyn LeRoy's 1929 film *Broadway Babies*. Economics, technology, and
the development of visual culture were all stacked against the Broadway
revue, but the new film musical would attempt—in grandiosity, production values, and style—to be honest-to-Ziegfeld.

Cinematic allusions to Ziegfeld abound in early musicals, beginning
with the stardom narrative *Broadway Melody* (Harry Beaumont, 1929).
This film is a particularly auspicious placement of the Ziegfeldesque because it was the first all-sound musical film and the prototype of its
genre, featuring the big production number, romantic backstage histri-
onics, and the gumption of the show-must-go-on hoofer.[9] The revue-
producer character in this film is the Great Zanfield, recognizable by
his trademark pickiness and lavishness, routinely spending two thousand dollars on an ermine cape that will be used for only ten minutes
onstage. Zanfield is the whimsical and all-powerful master of fate for
the narrative's protagonists, a small-town sister act arriving on Broadway for their big break. Zanfield first rejects them, then lets them into
the show, and finally determines at rehearsal that their skit is too slow
and replaces them with a chorus line. He decides to use Queenie (Anita
Page), the taller, blonder sister, as a tableau centerpiece, thus spelling the
end of the sister act. For the Zanfield tableau specialty, Queenie in her
beaded bra and loincloth simply stands on the prow of a ship, posing as
a masthead, above a crowd of Roman centurions and reclining, chiffon-
swathed slave girls. Although there is no direct reference in this film to
the Glorified American Girl, audiences in 1929 would have understood
that—as the taller, blonder preference—Queenie had instantly attained
the zenith of chorus girl life: she had been Glorified.

The 1929 *Broadway Melody* also exemplifies the split between the Ziegfeld Girl as the mannequin-showgirl—yummy, statuesque Queenie—

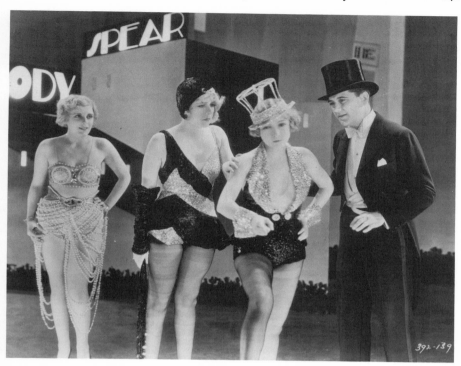

Anita Page is Queenie, the taller blond in the middle, who is the glorified girl in *Broadway Melody* (1929). (The Museum of Modern Art/Film Stills Archive)

and as the talented singer and dancer, her spunky sister Hank (Bessie Love). Since 1914 the Ziegfeld enterprise had promoted the former as its distinguishing icon, at the same time pumping the careers of its genuinely talented Follies Girls—Marilyn Miller, Mary Eaton, Ann Pennington—who were performers rather than fashion mannequins. The two kinds of revue girls show up again in *Ziegfeld Girl*, with similar splits in the narrative. By the closure of *Broadway Melody*, Queenie is married and retired from the stage, whereas Hank, hooked up with a new blond, is booked on another circuit and is on the road once more, praised as a "born trouper." In a larger cultural logic behind the wife-or-showgirl paradigm, being a wife makes sense for the luscious Queenie as the "real woman" of the pair. Hank's career also "makes sense" in that it de-

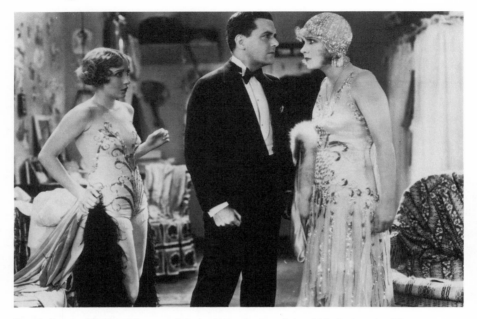

Bessie Love, Charles King, and Anita Page in *Broadway Melody* (1929). (The Museum of Modern Art/Film Stills Archive)

fines the career girl as young, attractive, and working in short skirts for the pleasure of men. The glamour is undeniably Queenie's; the appeal and sincerity of Hank are something else. The "something else" is immediately identifiable, in retrospect, as the quality Judy Garland would bring to nearly identical characters in film musicals (and in *Ziegfeld Girl*), in which she is the born trouper, the triumphant but vulnerable showbiz kid outside the cookie-cutter machine of traditional heterosexual appeal.

These splits and ambiguities of the ideal revue showgirl are breezily avoided in the 1929 film adaptation of *Sally,* certainly the most fairy-tale version of all Ziegfeld Girl film narratives. Both *Sally* and *Rio Rita,* musicals originally produced by Ziegfeld onstage, were box office cinema hits that year, with *Sally* attracting special attention because it featured its Broadway star Marilyn Miller, the Ziegfeld Girl closely identified as the Cinderella/Sally character. In the plotline, the heroine takes advantage of a mistaken identity to join the high-society crowd, find romance, and be discovered as a dancer. As the most recent Ziegfeld history points out, *Sally's* mistaken-identity theme suggests some of the illusions and superficial appearances bound up in the pursuit of the American Dream. But the Ziegfeld trademark as deus ex machina closes down whatever ambiguities cling to *Sally's* lighthearted escapades. At the end of the film, the heroine's problems are shelved when a friend arrives with a contract for the *Ziegfeld Follies:* "This fellow Ziggy is crazy about you!" [10] In the final five minutes of screen time, Sally rises out of a giant tulip onstage in her ballerina costume, resolves her romantic dilemma, and makes her triumphant appearance as a bride in the arches of a magnificent church. The closing marriage shots take place in a lush setting that could easily be one of the *Follies'* wedding-theme numbers, so that the *Follies'* production of sweet, domestic women and dazzling women stars is rendered as a seamless event.

In other films, the Ziegfeld legacy as a set of stylistic signs (the mannequin-showgirl, the headdresses and feathers, Busby Berkeley's sequined stagings of woman-as-decor) would have been instantly recognizable for audiences of this era with or without direct references to the *Follies* or Ziegfeld. Ziegfeld chronicler Randolph Carter speculates that even beyond the work of Berkeley, Ziegfeld's influence can be seen in Hollywood musicals well into the 1940s: "Except for King Vidor's *Hallelujah* and Robert Mamoulian's *Applause,* there is scarcely one of the scores produced that does not stem to some degree from Ziegfeld's concepts." Ziegfeld's concepts, at least the ones most adapted in cinema, were inevitably gendered concepts, the visual semantics of female bodies performing as patterns or designs for a presumed male camera/eye. [11]

The stylistics also point to the more complicated social and sexual issues with which the Ziegfeld enterprise was weighted after nearly thirty years of publicity and theater history. As even the brief description of *Broadway Melody* suggests, sexuality as well as gender is at stake in a narrative so adamant about breaking up a female team so that the "real woman" can be placed into a legitimate marriage. [12] The very stagings of "real women" in the Zanfield/Ziegfeld revue illustrate a need to align bodies, costumes, and desires into coherent definitions. Similarly, larger cultural issues are implied in the film musical "exceptions" named by Randolph Carter; in *Applause* (1929) the showgirl is part of the lower-class burlesque circuit, whereas *Hallelujah* (1929) is renowned as the best early musical film featuring a black cast. That is, Ziegfeld's stylistic concepts, borrowed by cinema, were organized not only by gender and sexual categories but by class and racial ones as well.

The power of the Ziegfeld showgirl as cultural icon is revealed in the way certain identities and values are conflated in these films — the showgirl as the unquestionably preferred display; tall, blond Queenie as the masthead and later the ideal mother/wife. Because the associations and meanings of the Ziegfeld Girl remained in public culture during the developing years of the Hollywood musical film, they constitute a significant contextual discourse, to use Janet Staiger's terms, an interpretive reading grid that would have been available to contemporary audiences of these films.[13] For current film studies, this context offers a way to understand how a specific cultural history — the Ziegfeld Girl — can be inscribed as a narrative structure and visual motif in a number of popular texts. In the larger context, these films constitute a small-scale demonstration of how a conservative ideology circulates and is reproduced in popular culture. As their appropriation in gay and camp culture illustrates, these images of the Ziegfeld Girl are contestable precisely because they are powerful; they are gist for marginalized comedy because they strain so earnestly to be mainstreamed.

What follows in this chapter are case studies of this contextual interpretation for three kinds of Hollywood musical films: (1) the two films Ziegfeld himself produced; (2) the two major biographical and historical tributes to Ziegfeld and his Girls; and (3) two early backstage musicals, choreographed by Busby Berkeley, which allude to the Broadway revue tradition. Ziegfeld's ventures in film production deserve attention not so much by virtue of their "Ziegfeld touch" — his input was actually minimal — but because they encapsulate some of the standardized connotations of the Ziegfeld Girl. *Glorifying the American Girl*, the awkward "perfect record" of Ziegfeld's revue, contains perhaps the only extant attempt to film an original *Follies* show. Far more interesting is *Whoopee!*, distinguished by the early work of Busby Berkeley and an astonishing performance by Eddie Cantor that led to more recent study of this film as an "Americanization" film based on racial masquerade.

The Great Ziegfeld and *Ziegfeld Girl,* as major MGM productions, are the popular texts that have most influentially carried the Ziegfeld trademark into cultural perpetuity. Both are concerned with stardom, one as a biopic and one as a generic reconstruction of the ideal Ziegfeld Girl. The irony of their Hollywood success is that they eagerly absorb the musical-theater milieu of Ziegfeld and flip-flop its implications, so that Hollywood cinema itself is glorified as the entertainment ideal. These two films also comparatively suggest the more complex social positioning of the Ziegfeld Girl as opposed to the positioning of Ziegfeld himself. The film biography of the famous showman avoids or shuts down ambiguity in order to posit him as artist-hero, streamlining the rough edges of his story into clear motivations and character traits. But the Ziegfeld Girl, given a film of her own, is diffused among three characters and contradictory visual and narrative elements, producing a far muddier composite showgirl. The issue of quality female talent versus commodified self-display, glossed over in *Broadway Melody,* is foregrounded and never easily resolved.

Finally, this chapter assesses two well-known backstage musicals, *Footlight Parade* and *Gold Diggers of 1933,* which do not directly reference Ziegfeld but which borrow from Ziegfeldian stylistics through the work of Busby Berkeley. As films of the depression, they offer a proliferation of female bodies as "riches," to use one well-known formulation, strikingly foregrounding the sexual and economic continuum of show business.[14] The Ziegfeld/Berkeley showgirl in these films also registers the contentions of racial whiteness and heterosexuality that, I have suggested, haunt the Ziegfeld project as its most obvious sites of definition and exclusion. Berkeley's over-the-top productions in these two films — women as gold coins, women as Anglo goddesses folding into waterfalls — choreograph these issues most dramatically as a direct cinematic inheritance from Ziegfeld's powerful theatrical tradition.

Ziegfeld Makes Movies

Ziegfeld hated Hollywood. All biographical accounts agree that, in spite of his marriage to film star Billie Burke, he saw cinema mostly as the rival entertainment that was stealing away his stars, just as he was known for stealing away the stars of rival shows. "Ziggy would have raised the scrubwoman's salary to keep her out of pictures," Louise Brooks said in an interview.[15] While the *Follies* operated as a display window for high-class fashion and other commodities, a 1932 fan magazine describes the *Follies* as a site where Hollywood directors went shopping—a "glittering show-window from which the shrewd motion picture magnate selects his hypnotic stars."[16]

Generally, the Ziegfeld Girls who would have an enduring reputation, the ones whose names are still fairly recognizable in popular culture, are the ones who succeeded in sound film: Ruby Keeler, Barbara Stanwyck, Louise Brooks, Paulette Goddard, Lina Basquette (via her connection with the Warner Brothers and her appearance as Cecil B. DeMille's godless girl), and Marion Davies—the last of whom haunts *Citizen Kane*. Because Marilyn Miller was the subject of a 1949 film (*Look for the Silver Lining*, David Butler), she too may have some current recognition value, though her 1985 biographer, Warren G. Harris, presents her with the expectation that pop culture does not remember "the other Marilyn."[17] Neither does it remember Olive Thomas, Mae Davis, Lillian Lorraine, and Ann Pennington, although these stars certainly occupy the "legendary realm" of the Ziegfeld Girl rhetoric. In spite of the brief careers many had in silent films, they have mostly been absorbed into the rubric of the Ziegfeld Girl.

The very maintenance of that rubric eventually outpriced itself. The production cost for Ziegfeld's 1932 show *Hot-Cha!* was close to half a million dollars, and when the show failed, he lost $115,000—a major blow for the depression era, especially in light of Ziegfeld's enormous losses in the 1929 crash. To the end, Ziegfeld insisted on the genuine article—the linen lining, the ostrich feather, the genuine fur, the real silk of the slipper. Most of all, he insisted on the "real" theatrical Ziegfeld Girl in the face of Hollywood cinema, claiming that "nothing will take the place of flesh and blood entertainment."[18] He paid his chorus girls higher-than-average salaries, and he was willing to outbid rival producers for stars. In the last years of the *Follies*, his chorus girls made $50 a week, his showgirls made up to $75, and Marilyn Miller got $3,680 a week for *Rosalie*—at a time when profits were generally falling for all Broadway shows.

In most other ways, Ziegfeld seems to have embraced the spirit of modernity; he loved telegrams, machinery, public relations—the "society of the spectacle," to use Guy deBord's term. But he failed to comprehend the long-term impact of mass reproduction, even though he himself ceaselessly reproduced versions of his Girl. Insisting on the individualized beauty of each showgirl, Ziegfeld counted on a public demand for her actual physical presence, as genuine as each rosette and ruby. He believed and invested in aura.

At one point Ziegfeld launched a pugnacious ad campaign against cinema, emphasizing the value of physical presence: "Ziegfeld *Follies*— Glorifying the American Girl in the Flesh—Not Canned." But after his serious losses in the market crash of 1929, Ziegfeld went to Hollywood, entered a partnership with Samuel Goldwyn, and in a number of press releases explained his plans to film a series of musical revues. Each interview emphasized that this was only a sideline to his "real" work on Broadway. "I will produce the genuine 'Follies' in sound pictures and show up all imitations," one such interview asserted, referring to the number of competing Broadway revues that used the same formula and often a version of the same name. But he was also concerned with the imitation of Hollywood cinema itself. "My 'Follies' girls alone will make the record a masterpiece with their beauty, for they are the real and only glorified girls. I will spend $3,000,000 to make my Movietone of 'Follies' the perfect record of the perfect revue that has so many ineffective imitators."[19]

His promised cinematic documentation, a "perfect record" of "the real and only glorified girls," became *Glorifying the American Girl*, three years in the making, with Ziegfeld involved with the story line as early as 1925. The film is so slow and visually boring that it bombed in 1929 as that year's "musical equivalent of *Ishtar*," as one film historian has put it.[20] Straining to use the camera as the position of the ideal *Follies* spectator— in effect, reverting to the theater—*Glorifying* stubbornly refuses its own premises, obstinately insisting that nothing will take the place of flesh-and-blood entertainment. The film's tedious pace seems to bank on an audience's unwavering fascination with a Glorified Girl in the making. Wholly without suspense, the narrative follows a fated-to-be-glorified young woman (yes, actually named Gloria) from department store clerk-dom to a brief vaudeville career to immediate success in Ziegfeld's *Follies*.

Nevertheless, as Paramount's opportunity to cash in on the Ziegfeld trademark and mythology, *Glorifying the American Girl* suggests some of the cultural implications of "Ziegfeld's concepts," especially in the gendered organization of commodification and work and in the organization of the female spectacle scenes as dreamy, nearly surreal displays. Busby Berkeley would later exploit this kind of spectacle as cinematic fantasy, but *Glorifying* provides a glimpse of its theatrical origins and also a glimpse of its wider social dynamics.

The narrative's one-track progress, from department store to *Follies* revue, links these two institutions, so that Gloria's middle-class occupation in the world of display showcases is a stepping-stone to the high-class showcase of the Ziegfeld revue. Remarkably, the narrative does not repeat the Ziegfeld fairy tale of *Sally*, in which stardom is rewarded by a happy closure and marriage, but goes the route that would eventually be made classic by Hollywood versions of *A Star Is Born:* female stardom means personal misery and sacrifice. Although Eddie Cantor supplies comedy in his stage act in the final reels, the film's story of Gloria's rise, discovery, and glorification is totally, dryly, relentlessly devoid of humor, having excised the possibility of female comedy by not including the extremely popular Fanny Brice, who was, along with Cantor, one of Ziegfeld's biggest stars. *Glorifying* is simply not interested in Brice's variety of less glamorous female stardom.

Granted, the sad story line of *Glorifying* is generally played down in deference to the musical interludes and spectacles. Yet even the spectacle or entertainment numbers repeat the dynamic of female stardom as a passive rather than an active, positive force. The sense of "show" for women consists of floating and twirling in magnificent display cases, whereas "show" for men involves the world of business, transaction, argument, and wit. As a carryover from the organization of the Broadway *Follies*, *Glorifying* calls on the Jewish comedy of Eddie Cantor for contrast to the showgirls in the film. Cantor plays comic relief, but he also provides the ethnic background against which the meaning of the showgirls comes into relief.

Cantor's comedy skit is the break between two musical-spectacle numbers: Gloria's dancing debut and the grand finale, "Loveland," a tribute to the *Follies'* famous "Laceland" production, glorifying little

Gloria as featured Ziegfeld star. The women's costuming in both big numbers includes chic evening gowns, ballet tutus, sequined pajamas, and outlandish attire that turns women into giant swans, butterflies, and flowers. A few groups of women wear matching costumes, but many of the more elegant and more outrageous gowns are unique, presenting amazing variety along the theme of feathers and sequins. Moving among the intricate staging, the women match the columns and bric-a-brac, blending into the architecture—the "living curtain" effect—so the result is not just fetishization but a literalization of women as decor. If you look carefully at "Loveland," you can see a few men who occasionally parade with a female partner to thematize the piece, but their costumes—flowing robes that trail behind them for several feet—are so feminized that it is difficult to sort them out in the claustrophobically jammed mise-en-scène. The final "glorification" shots of the film are close-ups of Gloria accepting applause and struggling with her feelings for a moment (her old boyfriend has just married The Nice Brunette) before realizing the absolute joy and supremacy of her triumph (Ziegfeld costuming and showcasing).

The Eddie Cantor skit that punctuates these two numbers is also focused on clothing. The setup is Moe the Tailor with a harassed customer, and in contrast to the two spectacle numbers, men's clothing is brashly demystified and placed in the context of business and work. In the course of the skit, men's jackets are ripped, chalked up, argued over, measured, altered, tried on, and destroyed. As opposed to the infinite, luxurious variety represented in the women's numbers, men's clothing here looks fairly standardized and utilitarian. Moreover, clothing is a product and part of a business in this number—specifically, a business in a Jewish neighborhood, designated by two signs in the background for "Solomon Klutz" and "Marcus Lipsitz." The ethnic specificity associated with Cantor foregrounds the importance of Gloria Hughes's blond non-ethnicity, further reinforced by her mother's British accent, the overwhelming whiteness of the women's costumes, and the silent black maid who attends her in the backstage scene.

Granted that clothing sales were in fact organized along gendered lines at this time, all three of these *Follies* numbers position women as mannequins and men as active shoppers and salesclerks, a dynamic that clearly contradicts how American women functioned as active, public consumers by 1929. As opposed to the social specificity of the Cantor routine, the female spectacle numbers look like hallucinations, utterly unattached to narrative, place, or time. Gloria's "glorification," her exalted position on the pedestal framed in her headdress and surrounded by sparkling and feathered women, is her abstraction into terms the Ziegfeld enterprise took seriously: sumptuousness, elegance, and, of course, pulchritude.

In the world organized by this sequence of *Follies* numbers, men are consumers and workers who argue, negotiate, joke, and complain in a recognizable real-life public place (the garment district). By withdrawing women from that historical world and placing them in a surreal "Love-land," this sequence denies even a very conservative idea of women as ideal consumers during the 1920s, situating women in "love," far outside of the active world of shopping and working. Clothing and work are mystified at their very site in the dressing room backstage, in fact, in which a pampered Gloria is coifed and headdressed with sacramental reverence, a clear contrast to the cheerful constructions and deconstructions of men's clothing in the Cantor skit. "Fashion" in this case instructs a passive, sex-segregated female behavior actually associated with a previous era, constructing a body that can display pleasurable scenarios only for others.

Women's costuming and fashion in these numbers evokes an oddly Victorian, sex-segregated world apart from the world of employment and work. As Charles Affron has said of the Ziegfeldian showgirl image in cinema, the woman is "subservient to an absurd costume that is not a dress, that is difficult to wear, that makes her top-heavy and/or bottom-heavy, that weighs her down and must be carried up."[21] Affron's point is that womanhood as adult sexuality is oddly denied in such images; larger cultural ideals about modern womanhood are denied as well, in a nostalgia for the woman weighed down into her role and clothes.

This nostalgia cues the film in the striking opening montage sequence, in which secretaries, laundresses, and dishwashers are magically glorified, their working clothes transformed into stunning evening gowns and headdresses. If we read this opening against the closing sequence of numbers, we can see a nostalgic wish for young white women to leave the workplace altogether to be part of a more abstract order of femininity, "glorified" through Ziegfeld's "processing."

The opening montage also cues the racial implications of glorification. The transformed young women are first seen as miniature figures on a superimposed map of the United States, marching toward New York in white robes — an image that, by 1930, when the Klan was actually making its own films, is not entirely innocent even if entirely guileless. Like the general Ziegfeld project, *Glorifying the American Girl* naturalizes the white body-for-show as an inevitable class distinction and commodity value. Mary Eaton as the ultimate, frothy vision of Ziegfeldness begins as the department store public blond, associated with valuable wares. When she makes the class move to the *Follies*, she acquires the African American maid to complete the meaning of her own value as preferred public body — or the "standardized" Ziegfeld body, to use the terms of Ziegfeld publicity at this time.

The theme of the racially acceptable female body is far more foregrounded in Ziegfeld's only other direct association with cinema, *Whoopee!* (Thornton Freeland, 1930), coproduced with Samuel Goldwyn as an adaptation of the 1928 Ziegfeld Broadway hit. *Whoopee!*'s narrative concerns a white girl's prohibited marriage to a man who is partly Native American. The last-minute plot device reveals that he is actually a well-tanned white man, adopted at birth by the tribe, so the couple can unite in the good spirit of romantic comedy. The flimsy plotline — actually a parody of a number of American frontier chestnuts — is mostly an excuse for the zany Eddie Cantor comedy and smart production numbers. Busby Berkeley's choreography reveals the editing and framing styles that would become his signature: the overhead shot turning bodies into geometric patterns and the tracking shot through the legs of chorus girls. Martin Rubin points out that this was Berkeley's first such use of these devices in cinema and firmly establishes Berkeley's films in the "Ziegfeldian stage tradition."[22]

The Ziegfeldian stage tradition is also inscribed in this musical as the boundary between the comedy and the showgirl spectacles, and the transgressions of the former as a measure of the high stakes of the latter. True to the Ziegfeld revue structure, the white showgirl body (and its version as the heroine imperiled by interracial flirtation) is set up as a contrast to the ethnic skits of Cantor. Cantor's outrageous behavior in this film boldly acts out numerous racial, social, and sexual transgressions that undermine any kind of stable identity but also stop short of sullying the status of the white American Girl body.

Cantor is cast as Henry Williams, the feminized, Jewish, hypochondriac pal of the romantic leads. As a city dude wholly out of place in the Wild West, Henry Williams is also wholly out of place in a heterosexual plotline. This familiar vaudeville persona is what Mast calls "Cantor's defining himself as a woman among men."[23] Much of the comedy involves his avoidance of the assertive, romantically inclined ranch nurse as he tries to help the "true" romantic couple unite. But Cantor plays gay even in scenes when the ranch nurse is not present, kissing the sheriff on the cheek and teasing the American Indian braves. He giggles and admires the shirtless physique of the male romantic lead, and he flirts openly with a warrior who has addressed him in a native language. "Aren't we all?" Cantor leers to him coyly in reply, chucking him under the chin.

Cantor's persona in this film is unabashedly queer—that is, performative, improvisational, resistant to any stable identity, sexual or racial. Alternately Orthodox Jewish, blackface, and redface, it also shifts between lecherous impulses toward anything female and fawning advances toward macho cowboys and American Indian warriors. While the narrative humorlessly defines the white, heterosexual couple and approves their marriage, Cantor enacts a reckless disruption of boundaries in a series of comic skits, many of which are as entirely dislocated from the romantic plot as the elaborate Busby Berkeley numbers. As critics have pointed out, Cantor's wild, transgressive comedy effectively mocks the text's nervousness about whom white girls should marry.[24]

Yet the film is also crazily split in its agendas, with the irreverent, carnivalesque work of Cantor totally disjointed from the text's more careful deference toward the white heroine and her showgirl clones. Michael Rogin places *Whoopee!* within a group of "Americanization" films that play with mobile identities and racial masquerade to emphasize the shared whiteness of European immigrants and hence their ability to be assimilated, to be Americans. Rogin reminds us that *Whoopee!*'s exclusions are still race-specific; its comic fluidity is limited to Cantor's Jewish performance and stops at the point of actually admitting black or

American Indian self-expression and identity.[25] More than that, the one solid identity audiences of 1930 would not have missed was the Ziegfeld showgirl as decor in Berkeley's opulent chorus displays.

The most serious—and hence, for today's viewers, perhaps the oddest—moments of *Whoopee!* put both comedy and narrative on hold so that forty showgirls could parade toward the camera in fluffy, elaborate bridesmaids dresses or in the svelte, peekaboo evening gowns of the finale. The Girl spectacles are demarcated from Cantor's performances even when they share the same space, so Ziegfeld Girls pose flirtatiously in wedding-attendant gowns behind Cantor's serious singing of the title song, apparently not comprehending its cynicism about marriage. While most other elements in this film are parodied—the macho cowboy, the wealthy ranch owner, the adopted-at-birth narrative—the fashion displays are positioned utterly without irony—like the serious "glorification" language Gilbert Seldes heard in the Ziegfeld offices. Situated among the more playful masquerades and ethnic/racial disguises of *Whoopee!* is the Glorified American Girl as a "genuine" article, a real boundary of "Americanization," that could make possible a liminal space for Cantor's clowning.

This dynamic is most evident in the film's revelation sequence, in which the American Indian suitor discovers his real parentage and hence ends the plotline's flirtation with a racially mixed marriage. This scene is introduced by two numbers that are ostensibly irrelevant to the plotline: a Cantor routine and an elegant Ziegfeldesque showgirl production. Both skits work on the principle of a masquerade lifted away to reveal a "true" identity. In the comedy routine, Cantor/Henry Williams is in double disguise as an Indian chief, complete with headdress, but in the persona of Jewish Moe the Tailor, trying to sell a blanket and Indian doll to a white man. The ever vigilant ranch nurse is the one who sees through all the disguises and tries to collar the hapless Henry. Without transition, the next shot begins the grand finale, the Ziegfeldian parade of Indian princesses, which also involves a revelation of identity. The showgirls make a stately entrance in procession wrapped in American Indian blankets and wearing Indian-style feathered headdresses; as each showgirl nears the camera, she lifts away the blanket to reveal a stunning 1930s-style evening gown beneath.

In contrast to the previous comedy skit, which had likewise lifted away disguises to reveal an identity—Henry Williams beneath the Indian chief and Moe the Tailor—the fashion-show spectacle is carried out in a tone of sober awe. Henry Williams and his multilayered racial and sexual masquerades are funny fantasies, but the film insists on a more stable white, female body. The Indian procession is immediately recognizable as a fashion-show parade, the rocky Western landscape becomes a fashion-show ramp, and in 1930, the mannequin/showgirls would have been instantly seen to be Ziegfeld Girls. Confirming this, a second legion of showgirls enters on horseback, each wearing huge feather headdresses and nude-colored jeweled bra and panties. After the ensemble lines up for a Ziegfeld-style tableau, the *Whoopee!* plotline continues, with the Indian suitor discovering his real racial identity. As in the showgirl performance, white culture is "saved" after a flirtation with transgression, the trademark showgirl providing a visualization of the status quo.

This grand production number of the Indian-turned-Ziegfeld Girl also works in the logic of café au lait blackface. The elaborate feathered American Indian headdresses "pass" as the famous showgirl headdresses of the Ziegfeld stage. The headdress is a fantasy fetishization of another culture and race—a denial of its difference, an encompassing of its threat. In combination with the nude effect on horseback—a nude effect that is actually decidedly non-Indian jeweled underwear—this Ziegfeld masquerade sums up the desires for both whiteness and an exotic racial Other: desire for the "authentic" or natural female body but also the desire to decorate and fetishize it into a magnificent commodity with a readable price tag.

Without doubt, the pleasure of the film is Cantor's performance, a perverse and polymorphous fantasy. But the other fantasy of this film, one that makes possible Cantor's bizarre marginality, is the specificity of the Ziegfeld Girl as a tease of forbidden desires packaged in a safe, recognizable iconography. As the white, heterosexual, bourgeois body, she is the mannequin modeling what Americans are supposed to look like, the "real" American in a mélange of cartoons.

Stardom: The Great Ziegfeld *and* Ziegfeld Girl

The power and powerful contradictions of Ziegfeld's showgirl as a "type" are most evident in the film that secured her name forever in popular culture, Robert Z. Leonard's 1941 *Ziegfeld Girl*. This is especially noticeable in contrast to *The Great Ziegfeld*, the more straightforward stardom film honoring the producer himself. Long before his death in 1932, Ziegfeld's publicity office and popular journalism had constructed Ziegfeld not just as consummate producer and artistic master but as hero and star as well. The titles of Cantor and Freedman's 1934 biography, *Ziegfeld, the Great Glorifier*, and the 1936 MGM biopic, *The Great Ziegfeld*, the first two major posthumous biographical texts, thus fittingly characterize Ziegfeld as a larger-than-life legend. For readers and audiences of the 1930s, these titles would also have resonated as allusions to F. Scott Fitzgerald's 1925 best-selling novel *The Great Gatsby* and its hero, the gorgeous if doomed entrepreneur who, like the Ziegfeld persona, remained a powerful but mysterious presence behind splendid scenarios and gestures.

Like Gatsby, Ziegfeld ended his career in disarray rather than glory. The Ziegfeld musicals *Show Boat*, *Rio Rita*, *Rosalie*, and *Whoopee!* were major hits during the 1927 and 1928 seasons, but the *Follies* revues had peaked and were in decline, the formulas overfamiliar and the expenditures out of control. Ziegfeld's 1929 *Show Girl*, the stage version of J. P. McEvoy's popular novel, was a disaster, and other production disasters followed, including the phenomenal box office failure of the *Glorifying the American Girl* film. Even the financial success of the film version of *Whoopee!* did not earn Ziegfeld enough to keep him financially viable. When he died in 1932—ironically, in Hollywood rather than in his beloved theater town New York—he was between three hundred thousand and five hundred thousand dollars in debt, and he had just a little under three thousand dollars in cash to his name.[26]

In spite of this sad ending and probably because the depression had made financial misery a commonplace, Ziegfeld's death brought him immediate canonization in show business history and in the public domain. Some of the newspaper eulogies specifically glamorized him in Gatsby-like terms; he "seemed to live in a dream of splendor beyond count or cost," the *New York American*'s drama critic effused. The *New York Times* obituary struck a similar note, re-creating the Ziegfeld persona as a mystery, the source of his "magic" difficult to track down and "hard to define."²⁷ The characterizations as magician, dream master, and mystery man were not simply posthumous romanticizations but also qualities that had been cultivated by Ziegfeld publicity for decades.

For much of his career, Florenz Ziegfeld was a "character" in popular culture, the focus of theater anecdotes, rumors, and his own press releases. His romantic involvement with Anna Held and his prominence as a big spender in the New York theater scene had secured him celebrity by the turn of the century. Later, his reputation grew with that of his annual revues, so feature articles were likely to emphasize "Ziegfeld of the 'Follies' and the way in Which He Glorifies the American Girl." The mystiques of authorship, success, conspicuous consumption, and association with showgirls drew curiosity about the details of his personal life and management style. Soon, Ziegfeld was posited as a colorful public image behind which lay a "set of secrets . . . beneath a set of secrets, *en abyme,*" to use Richard deCordova's terms. This public image played successfully to what Raymond Williams would call the era's "structure of feeling": an exuberant embrace of commodification; showcase opulence, and admiration of wealth and of the era's captains of industry.²⁸

Soon after Ziegfeld's 1914 marriage to Billie Burke, one of his publicity writers published an insider's scoop shamelessly claiming the marriage itself was timed to get headlines away from a sensationalized execution at Sing Sing and succeeded in doing so. Like other Ziegfeld personality sketches at this time, this article also calls attention to the lush personal extravagance that matched the extravagance of Ziegfeld's theatrical style. "Mr. Ziegfeld wants what he wants when he wants it, and he usually finds a way to get it. All of Mr. Ziegfeld's wants are costly." Rumors were pumped that he never wore the same suit twice, for example, and that he casually hired personal chefs and barbers on whims. This particular article references Ziegfeld's horses, yacht, and yachting clothes—"a change of apparel for each shift of wind."²⁹ Commodity consumption is not just celebrated here but explicitly admired as one of his talents. The description of the clothing, moreover, strongly rhymes with the kind of high-fashion discourse used to describe the clothing displays in the *Follies*, so that Ziegfeld is imagined as part of the spectacles he was producing. The tone of the essay makes it clear that by 1914, Ziegfeld himself was a celebrity and star.

Other Ziegfeld press releases characterized his micromanagement style as captain-of-industry heroism. "It has always been a mystery, even to his intimates, how this manager of unfailing resource could accomplish all the myriad details of his work," one such story ran. "The answer is 'by concentration and invention.' In every waking hour this trim, athletic, fastidiously groomed young man keeps his alertly inventive mind working like a machine gun." Another story quotes the Ziegfeld persona boasting of this obsessiveness: "It's detail that counts. If I've made a success with my eight consecutive *Follies* and my other musical comedies it's because I've watched details." Ziegfeld was also characterized as ascetically detached, in spite of his persistence and drive. "But presuming Mr. Ziegfeld really possesses emotions," one story ran, "he is singularly reticent about expressing them. His demeanor is remarkably even under widely varying conditions. He stands a loss and takes a profit with equal apparent equanimity."[30] On the one hand, this characterization is straight out of Horatio Alger fiction ("concentration and invention"); on the other hand, the tone of awe reminds us that Ziegfeld was lionized in the era of the mogul (a "manager of unfailing resource"). As a "captain of industry," Ziegfeld was the entertainment business's equivalent of a Henry Ford, J. P. Morgan, or Randolph Hearst: enormously successful and greatly publicized. Not surprisingly, the Ziegfeld persona in the press releases often cites his own heroism in epic terms, if in mixed metaphors: "I recently picked out . . . forty-four of the most beautiful chorus girls in America. It was a labor of Hercules, going over the whole chorus girl crop of 1914 with a fine-toothed comb."[31]

One of the favorite self-promotions of the Ziegfeld enterprise was its absolute modernity and its leadership in Ziegfeld as twentieth-century genius. He loved the inventions of the telephone and telegraph, using them for publicity stunts, business, and personal relationships. Contemporary feature stories emphasized this fascination: "He has several telephones at his bedside, and starts the day by a liberal use of them. He never writes letters, he says, and the telegraph and telephone take their place." [32] Multiple stories confirm Ziegfeld would regularly send a telegram from the back of the theater to someone up onstage. His wife Billie Burke good-humoredly but realistically complained, in a telegram answering his, that "ITS [sic] TOO BAD WE NEVER TALK THINGS OVER EXCEPT WITH THE WESTERN UNION." [33] When the first transatlantic radio phone service was made available in 1927, Ziegfeld managed to be the first to call London. [34] The interest in gimmicks was allied to the publicity gimmicks and stagecraft. As an industrialist of female bodies, Ziegfeld was fascinated with the interaction of body and machine, body and gimmick; his acts were full of cleverly designed rotating stages, lighting systems, moving platforms, and, of course, the choreographed body. The Cantor and Freedman biography incorporates these well-known Ziegfeldian quirks into the book's hype; the "three great inventions" of the twentieth century, it asserts, are "the telephone, the telegraph, and the American Beauty — and Florenz Ziegfeld was the leading exponent of all three." [35]

While the personal details of clothing, yachting, and communication gimmicks were carefully delivered to the public, Ziegfeld publicity also set up his theatrical success as a "mystery" and tied it to the "mystery" of Ziegfeld's personality. "He steals in and out of the theater without anyone knowing that 'Ziggy' has been around," one such story claimed. Ziegfeld's solitude, according to this press release, "enables him to cloak his own personality and activities in a kind of picturesque mystery." In published interviews the Ziegfeld persona often concurs in this: "I am carried away with the mystery and thrill" of show business success, one such story immodestly begins. [36] Perhaps as a legacy of this public image, the connotation of unknowability continued in a number of later representations of Ziegfeld — in films such as *Ziegfeld Girl*, for example, where his sacred presence is wholly off-camera, or in *The Will Rogers Follies*, in which the voice of "Ziegfeld" calls out from darkness at the back of the theater.

The quality of being unknowable reinforced and justified Ziegfeld's position as one-who-knows — that is, as a professional judge of women's faces and bodies. The godlike persona made possible the mainstream expertise I described in Chapter 4. "Where on earth does Ziegfeld get them every year? Such an array of peach orchard, blossoming beauties." [37] This imagination of Ziegfeld as the Genesis creator in his garden, combined with the discourse on his "mystery" (what is he really like?), created the overall effect of the superior, invisible observer. Rick Altman, pointing out the considerable influence of Ziegfeldian theater on film musicals, describes the dynamic as: "woman as image, man as voice." [38] One of the specific sources of this dynamic is this previous Ziegfeld public persona as an apparatus of surveillance, a judge and measurement of women's bodies—not just a generalized "male gaze" but a concrete one, with a public relations voice speaking in interviews and press releases.

Given these previous decades of lionization, the Ziegfeld public persona was well primed for Hollywood characterization in 1936, with specifically Gatsby-like glamour. In *The Great Ziegfeld,* the romantic charm of Jay Gatsby is reinscribed as Ziegfeld's ability to enthrall Anna Held, to capture the heart of Billie Burke, and to have a blond, long-legged beauty (obviously based on Lillian Lorraine) at his call. Gatsby as dreamer and impossible idealist is reworked as Ziegfeld the lover of loveliness and the perfectionist showman. The Gatsby who glimpsed the ladder "to a secret place above the trees" [39] becomes the Ziegfeld whose dying words are "Higher! Higher!"—directions to long-gone stage crews and exclamations of his own ambition and aesthetic.

Ziegfeld's milieu was in fact part of the social scene referenced in *The Great Gatsby.* The understudy of Gilda Gray—the real-life *Follies* star who sang "Getting Darker" in 1922—supposedly shows up at one of Gatsby's grandiose parties. As suggested by the presence of the understudy rather than the star herself, Fitzgerald's extensive list of VIPs at Gatsby's house is pointed and cynical: "the Hornbeams and the Willie Voltairs, and a whole clan named Blackbuck, who always gathered in a corner and flipped up their noses like goats at whosoever came near. And the Ismays and the Chrysties (or rather Hubert Auerbach and Mr. Chrystie's wife)." [40] In the New York newspapers Fitzgerald knew quite well, press releases regularly announced the stellar presences in the audience at Ziegfeld shows: the Hearsts, the Astors, Governor Alfred E. Smith, Mayor James Walker, Mr. and Mrs. S. Hutton, Jerome Kern, Maurice Chevalier, Bernard Baruch, Bernard Gimbel, George S. Kaufman, Diamond Jim Brady. As one theater critic put it, the audience typically included "practically everybody known on Broadway who is not in Europe or in a hospital." [41]

That is, the class markers of the Ziegfeld shows were its audiences

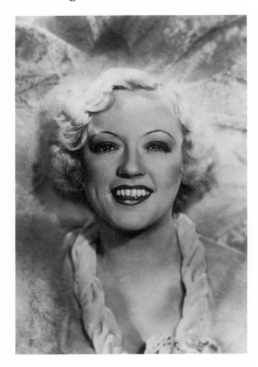

Marion Davies, the Ziegfeld star and later film star whose career was orchestrated by Randolph Hearst. (Billy Rose Theatre Collection, New York Public Library for the Performing Arts)

as much as its high-fashion spectacles, its ability to draw "everybody known on Broadway." As Jay Gatsby carefully calculated, mere association was enough to earn privilege and respect. In the Fitzgerald novel, the mix of would-be celebrities and old and new money constitutes both puffy posturing and real power; Gatsby was the imaginative creation of Jimmy Gatz, but within his circle of influence, we are told, the World Series was fixed in 1919.

Prominent Ziegfeld audience member Randolph Hearst was a friend of Ziegfeld's who would himself make former Follies Girl Marion Davies a star. He forms part of a significant triad here because in the long run, the fictional Jay Gatsby haunts the fictionalizations of both Hearst and Ziegfeld. In this association of wealthy men, Hearst, Ziegfeld, and Gatsby are notable for creating magnificent spectacles and *performing* their wealth to the delight of a curious public. For all three, the mystery of personality is heightened by their sensationalized discourse (yellow journalism, "How I Pick My Beauties," rumors of murder and gang-sterism) and dazzling images (San Simeon, *Follies* tableaux, the cream-colored Rolls Royce).

The Fitzgerald novel reveals the moral bankruptcy of creating iden-tity as image, its haunting title sheathed in irony. Eventually Orson Welles would capture that irony by rewriting Gatsby as Randolph Hearst in *Citizen Kane,* suggesting a controversial life of excess, mystery, and contradictions.[42] When the young Charles Kane steals the writing staff of the rival newspaper (like Ziegfeld's theft of stars from rival shows), the celebratory fete features leggy showgirls who form a kicking, sing-ing background for Kane himself as ringmaster and star. Later, the older Kane, more producer than star, steps backstage to manipulate and man-age fascist politics, on the one hand, and the coerced performances of Susan Alexander, on the other. Kane's erection of an entire theater for Susan's performances may have referenced the stunning Ziegfeld The-ater that Hearst financed for Ziegfeld in 1926, a building that was itself a monument to Ziegfeldian expansiveness and showiness.

Both *The Great Gatsby* and *Citizen Kane* in the end emphasize the un-readable nature of men who invest in breathtaking public display as self-representation; the empty Xanadu and the deserted Gatsby mansion are museums rather than personal signatures, and at the conclusions of the Fitzgerald novel and the Welles film, the observer can only back away with riddles instead of answers.

In contrast, Leonard's film *The Great Ziegfeld* offers an absolutely read-able and knowable Gatsby-like entrepreneur in Ziegfeld. After years of press releases touting him as a mystery, the biographical film just four years after his death seems like the solution to puzzles, a way of finally rendering him understandable. In the tradition of classic Hollywood cinema, every question or mystery is clarified rather than amplified. How did Ziegfeld get Anna Held from overseas? Charm. What kind of husband was he for Billie? Unswervingly devoted. How did he handle his financial losses? With pluck.

Writing about Hollywood biographical pictures, George F. Custen points out that the biopic is essentially self-serving to Hollywood's own interests and ideology. Thus *The Great Ziegfeld,* though supposedly cele-brating a life devoted to theater (and a career eventually threatened

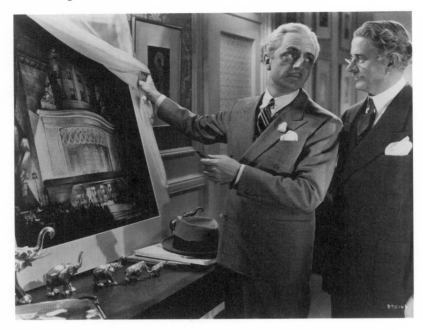

William Powell, left, as the title character of the film biography *The Great Ziegfeld,* 1936. (The Museum of Modern Art/Film Stills Archive)

by cinema), ends up acclaiming the superiority of the cinematic grand production number. The film also embodies the Ziegfeld persona in debonair William Powell, who essentially plays his sophisticated *Thin Man* character (1934)—unflappable, charming, bright—so the construction of Ziegfeld as star depends on recognition of another stardom and popular film. Reinforcing this connection is the casting of Myrna Loy, Powell's partner in *The Thin Man,* as Billie Burke. As Custen puts it, the biopic is "the star system speaking of itself." [43]

The Great Ziegfeld claims in its opening titles to be "suggested by romances and incidents in the life of America's greatest showman, Florenz Ziegfeld Jr." The "romances and incidents" are mostly the best-known Ziegfeld anecdotes from the previous decades: the fake milk bath, the financial recklessness, the ability to "steal" the stars from other revues. The film's reliance on audience knowledge is evident in an odd moment when William Powell's smooth Ziegfeld could be read, by the untutored viewer, as oddly effeminate. The first time we see him with an attractive woman, he tells her that her outfit of the day before, a red dress and a yellow hat, "was atrocious. Each was all right in itself, but in combination—whoooo!" "Aren't we the observer?" she replies sarcastically. Audiences of 1936 would immediately have recognized this not as effeminacy but as a clue about future fame: professional observation of women's clothing would become this man's career.

The film in this way deftly sums up a theme that showed up often in the published personality sketches of Ziegfeld during his lifetime: preoccupation with the details of women's clothing. "Nothing is too trivial to escape Mr. Ziegfeld's supervision. He personally selects and purchases every costume. He is responsible for every color scheme," one typical news story ran. The Ziegfeld persona voice adds, in the same piece: "I personally choose every hat that goes on every girl's head in my company." [44] Biographical sources suggest that the obsessiveness with his showgirls' fashions, hats, and fabrics, as represented in the press releases, had a real basis in Ziegfeld's personal style of management and production. Encoding this quality as genius deflects its more interesting overtones, particularly the implication that, as a well-known, dapper dresser himself, he identified with the women on display, as suggested by his "change of apparel for each shift of wind."

One of the earliest psychological theorists of fashion, J. C. Flugel, claimed in 1930 that men who need to "exhibit" women—to be seen publicly with beautiful or well-dressed women on their arms—are on some level identifying with the exhibited woman through "the projection of the exhibitionistic desire." Flugel's claim that men in Western culture had to "renounce" exhibitionist clothing at the end of the eighteenth century has been disputed, but the ubiquity of Ziegfeld's public persona as the observer of women and their clothing certainly suggests a male ego also "on show." [45]

The Great Ziegfeld, however, backs away from this possibility by imitating the dynamics of the *Follies* themselves, with great emphasis on the display of female bodies. The costuming greatly plays down Ziegfeld as exhibitionist, while every opportunity is taken to display the showgirl—fluffy, white, leggy, young. In this film, even the women characters who are not showgirls dress like showgirls, in oversize hats, elaborate gowns, and fitted costumes that call attention to breasts, waists, hips. Luise Rainer as Anna Held is constantly in bright dresses that seem sprayed onto her torso, flouncing out below the knees. William Powell as Ziegfeld, in contrast, wears dark suits that call no attention at all to his body and instead deflect attention to his head and the cravat at this throat: "woman as image, man as voice," to use Altman's phrase.

The one mystery *The Great Ziegfeld* strains to keep ambiguous is the sexual one. During his lifetime, Ziegfeld's constant references to "his girls" suggest a fatherly patronage, but they also suggest—as was certainly often true—that they were his girlfriends and lovers, an endless harem circulating around one powerful mogul. Although the Ziegfeld office presented the "fastidiously groomed young man" who "keeps his alertly inventive mind working like a machine gun," gossip columnists were eager to reveal his sexual scandals and adventures. Gorgeous, alcoholic Lillian Lorraine, one of his major romances during his relationship with Anna Held, was notorious for her public scenes that kept the columnists happy. Later, his fling with Olive Thomas brought rumors that Billie Burke was considering divorce. The later biographies admit that Ziegfeld's affairs with "his girls" were nearly continuous and probably escalated as he got older. In 1922, *Follies* star Marilyn Miller, with whom Ziegfeld was apparently obsessed if not romantically involved, gave an angry interview that made the *New York Times*, accusing Ziegfeld of "making love to chorus girls and of attempting to send [Miller] a diamond as big as her hand." If, as Richard deCordova suggests, sexual scandal is the "repressed underside" of the star system, this underside of the Ziegfeld persona as promiscuous lover was the knowledge both hidden and flaunted during his lifetime.[46] The substantial public affection for Held and later for Burke must have fueled the sexual curiosity, relentlessly reinforcing the truth of male privilege: he sleeps with his Girls.

This aura of sexual scandal presents a problem for *The Great Ziegfeld*. The Cantor and Freedman biography, a cleaned-up version of Ziegfeld's life, was absolutely silent about the sex scandals, but the authors conceded that Lillian Lorraine was "one of the very few [showgirls] to whom Zieggy was strongly attached." [47] The film version likewise acknowledges a relationship with a character named Audrey, a showgirl obviously representing Lorraine, probably because it was so widely known that the latter was greatly responsible for Anna Held's departure from Ziegfeld's life. Cantor and Freedman refrain from making this connection, but for the film biography, a clear cause had to be posited for the divorce from Held. Because Luise Rainer's Held is presented in such sympathetic terms, the film's problem is the presentation of the Audrey romance: how could Ziegfeld, star and hero, be engaged in a romance behind the back of his sweet (almost saintly) wife and still be star and hero?

As it turns out, the biopic's generic dependence on clear causality works previous to the Audrey plotline to set up the unfaithfulness. As Custen points out, biopics usually "explain fame through a specific motivating episode" that delineates the character of the famous person and illustrates the talent or genius that will single him or her out.[48] In this case, in an early episode at his father's house, Ziegfeld as a young man flirts with a precocious six-year-old music student, Mary Lou, explaining to her that she can't be "his girl" because he likes "*all* the girls. Some people like beautiful paintings. Some people love beautiful flowers. I love beautiful little girls." The rhetoric is echoed later in the film when Ziegfeld tells a nervous Anna, who has intuited his interest in the Lorraine character, "I'm interested in *all* my girls." The earlier little-girl scene may align this promiscuity with innocence and cuteness, but it also sets up an uncomfortable connotation of incest, a powerful "dance line daddy," to use Patricia Mellencamp's term, who is fond of "beautiful little girls."[49]

Mary Lou predictably shows up in his office twenty years later to be hired as a showgirl. But the latter scene is played purely for humor, with a discomfited Ziegfeld trying to wriggle out of the affectionate kisses of the grown-up "little girl." Generally, the rhyming episode reminds us that Ziegfeld's knack for loving "all the girls" accounts for his successful life as a revue producer—and, incidentally, his inclination toward unfaithfulness. Ironically, Marilyn Miller's biographer Warren G. Harris ascertains that Mary Lou was widely read as a version of Miller, who played a *jeune fille* in the *Follies* for years beyond her jeune-filleness.[50] As a female star who had to fight Ziegfeld's flirtations and jealousies, Miller is certainly ill served if her representation here serves to gloss over Ziegfeld's affairs with his other showgirls.

Generally, the casting and mise-en-scène also set up a causality for the Audrey romance. Luise Rainer, true to Anna Held's dimensions and coloring, is small and dark. Her French accent, French maid, and French voice teacher situate her in an enclave of exoticism in the New York nightclub scene. Virginia Bruce as Audrey, in contrast, is statuesque and blond. Audiences in 1936 would have had no trouble identifying the latter as a Ziegfeld Girl, if a scandalous one. Tough, brash, and boozy, Audrey is far from idealized, but she is a signal of the future — the Glorified American Girl who is tall, leggy, and light haired.

Moreover, Audrey marks the transition to second wife Billie Burke, fair-haired and all-American, as played by Myrna Loy. While Anna Held is fashioned as girllike, sweet, and quaint in a Victorian way, Billie is characterized as the confident modern woman, worldly and sophisticated. She tells Ziegfeld on meeting him that she hears he is a "terrible ladies man," but the implication is that, unlike the sweet Anna Held, tougher Billie will keep him out of trouble. So while the Audrey plotline gives us a cold glimpse of a philanderer showering his mistress with jewels and fur, the narrative embeds this within several public knowledges about Ziegfeld so that a logic of fame emerges: his extravagant spending, his estrangement from the European Anna Held, and his instinct to promote an "American type" of beauty all propel him to the position of "America's greatest showman."

Ziegfeld's more famous episodes of hype are reverently celebrated in this film. The Sandow promotion takes up the lengthy opening sequence, and discussion of the fake milk bath story comprises a major scene between Ziegfeld and Anna Held. Both episodes are constructed as tributes to the Ziegfeld genius, and as well-known, popular stories, they contribute to the illusion that the film gives us the "real" Ziegfeld, producer of spectacular theater and clever promotional tactics. The conflation of hype and entertainment gets naturalized as a way of understanding his success. In effect, his reputation as "the P. T. Barnum of the theater" structures the entire film, which opens with Ziegfeld literally as a carnival barker for Sandow and presents a circus-theme *Follies* number as its final musical production.

Deathbed scenes are especially meaningful capstones of the biopic, as Custen points out, a final "monumental depiction" of the film's subject.[51] *The Great Ziegfeld* generously resituates the showman's death in

New York, where he dies with a montage of various big production numbers superimposed on the screen, scores of dancers in elaborate costumes marching and swaying toward the camera. Ziegfeld's obituaries typically pointed out the number of comedians and musical performers made famous by the *Follies,* but this film insists that "beautiful little girls" are what Ziegfeld was about and that the big production number — exactly the kind of production number being staged for 1930s film musicals — was Ziegfeld's primary legacy. Considering the popularity of film musicals in the 1930s, especially Warner Brothers' Busby Berkeley style openly imitated in this MGM vehicle, the virtual canonization of Ziegfeld here acknowledges him as the origin of the glamorous, excessive 1930s cinematic musical number.[52] The film thus both celebrates and obfuscates the growing economic and cultural priority of films over Broadway musicals — a major reason we see Ziegfeld and his theater-producer friends equally broke in the final sequences.

The Great Ziegfeld's most spectacular and most often quoted production number is "A Pretty Girl Is Like a Melody," which epitomizes the Ziegfeldian legacy. This number features the Irving Berlin tune and a gigantic, circling wedding cake of a set, on which a winding staircase furnishes the display of a dazzling history of pretty girls, from minuet-dancing, eighteenth-century lasses to jazzy young women swaying to Gershwin tunes. While Busby Berkeley would have used dizzying editing to remove such a spectacle from realistic time and space, the filmmakers here aimed to be more true to the Ziegfeld elements of the staircase and a showgirl-as-scenery display. To achieve that effect but avoid the stilted, frozen ensemble of the actual Ziegfeld tableaux, the entire staircase set moves instead of the camera. The costumes of the showgirls vary dramatically, from puffy hooped skirts to catlike leotards, but the women seem identical, so that at one point a dozen matching heads bob in layers of tulle and chiffon. At the top of the wedding cake/spiral, the Audrey/Lillian Lorraine character holds court over the whole assemblage of bodies, the queen of blondness.

The lyrics sung by men in tuxedos assure us that a pretty girl is haunting, like a musical refrain. In addition, the visuals assure us that, as image, she is eternally the same Girl, the same universal body and face, with only costuming as a marker of history. That her universality

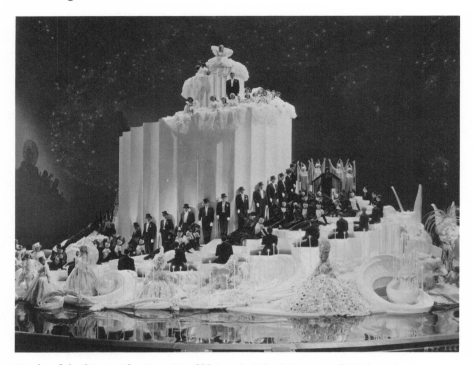

Finale of the biopic *The Great Ziegfeld* (1936). (The Museum of Modern Art/
Film Stills Archive)

is very narrowly defined—as young, white, blond, slender—is given
no ironic perspective. In *The Great Gatsby* and *Citizen Kane,* the adored
Daisy Buchanon and Susan Alexander are blond facades behind which
we glimpse an emptied-out culture. But the blond facades of the Girls
here, and later of the showgirl musical films, are meant to be appreciated as facades, "image of woman as image."

Reinforcing the general Ziegfeld mythology, the number "A Pretty
Girl Is Like a Melody" powerfully visualizes women as the raw material for male aesthetic vision and design. Womanhood in this production number is delineated as the fluffy, artificial tiers of costuming and
staging. *The Great Ziegfeld,* then, continues fairly seamlessly the adulat-
ing discourse Cantor and Freedman circulated in the *Ziegfeld* biography.
The Ziegfeld Girl herself was essentially raw material, they write, but

was transformed by Ziegfeld "in the magic of his [*sic*] clothes, the tint of his lights and the effect of his ensemble. . . . Glorifying the American girl was not merely a press agent's slogan—it was an actual process invented by Zieggy."[53]

The Ziegfeld material was still such hot copy in the early 1940s that MGM, with Leonard again as director, repeated the topic with *Ziegfeld Girl*, just five years after the highly successful, Academy Award–winning biopic. Although a focus on Ziegfeld had produced a fairly straightforward rising-star text, a focus on the Girl created a far more dissonant and interesting film. The clothes and "ensemble" of Ziegfeldness are, after all, the very fabric of gendered and racialized desires—the untanned skin, the discipline of the high-fashion Ziegfeld Walk, the genuine jewels and bourgeois body. Ziegfeld Girlhood, as this bundle of female ideals and frameworks, bristles with tensions and contradictions not easily resolvable through standard rise-from-the-chorus narratives.

Ziegfeld Girl could easily have gone this standard route as an updated *Sally*. The narrative of the talented chorus girl rising to stardom was familiar enough in cinema—for example, in *Show Girl in Hollywood* (1930), and *Blondie of the Follies* (1932). In its most popular 1930s form, this plotline featured a successful romance (a performing, talented, romantic couple) resulting in successful female stardom—*42nd Street* (1933), *Footlight Parade* (1933), and *Dames* (1934). However, plotlines about talent and merit are unworkable for a film featuring Ziegfeld's trademark showgirl-mannequin, who walked and wore clothes rather than performing a talent. "It is a little silly," the Hedy Lamarr character of *Ziegfeld Girl* tells her husband of her new showgirl position. "You just put on some beads or something and walk up and down." Moreover, unlike the Fred Astaire or Dick Powell character in earlier musicals who could envision, co-create, and coperform with his mate/musical partner, Ziegfeld himself could not be represented as such a cocreator without suggesting his embarrassing real-life romantic involvements with many of his showgirls.

To accommodate both terms of the title—privileged male artistry and a female story about self-display and commodification—*Ziegfeld Girl* worked within developments in the musical genre itself as well as within the complexity of the Ziegfeld cultural legacy. First, around this time the backstage musical began to take a more sharply self-conscious turn, emphasizing and critiquing specific problems in its own structure.[54] So the well-known commercial value of the Ziegfeld Girl, as a trademark product of Ziegfeld "processing" described in such detail by Cantor and Freedman and others, was foregrounded as an appeal to audience knowledge about the New York revue scene. The audition and backstage scenes in this film expose the competitive, coldly mechanical "business" of the *Follies*, especially as a business of sexual exchanges with men, and the Hedy Lamarr character dismisses the Ziegfeld Walk as "a little silly." Yet a few scenes after this remark is made, Ziegfeld glamour is wholly recuperated with the "You Stepped Out of a Dream" number in which showgirls are effortlessly lifted from male fantasy to "walk up and down" in a fabulous ensemble of costume and staging. In other words, the Ziegfeld enterprise as a well-known history and as a mystique reinforced the backstage formula of exposing but then re-glamorizing show business performances.[55]

Second, the generic Ziegfeld Girl of the film title is materialized by the conventions and plot devices of melodrama as much as by backstage formulas, in this way playing to audience expectations of "the woman's film" and also to preconceptions about Ziegfeld history. For 1941 audiences even remotely aware of show business gossip, melodrama would have been a particularly apt narrative mode and tone for the accumulated scandals and tragedies of well-known Ziegfeld Girls. Lillian Lorraine deteriorated due to heavy drinking and bankruptcy after her years on the Ziegfeld stage, and stories about her disruptive public appearances appeared in gossip columns for years. At a 1933 Ziegfeld tribute, she had left the stage in tears, unable to perform her scheduled song. *Follies* singer Ruth Etting made headlines in 1937 when her lover was shot by her former husband. Three years later, the spendthrift, millionaire-marrying *Follies* star Jessie Reed died a pauper and alcoholic. Olive Thomas died young of a drug overdose or poisoning, perhaps at the hands of her husband, Jack Pickford, who then married Ziegfeld's all-time golden girl, Marilyn Miller. In addition to her stormy relationship with Ziegfeld, Miller had previously suffered young widowhood, endured a bad marriage to Pickford, and died in 1936, at the age of thirty-five.

The appeal to this "real-life" history is stated outright early in the

film, when the backstage manager announces to the new *Follies* recruits
that the *Ziegfeld Follies* are "real life, but faster." Some of them, he pre-
dicts, will wind up as stars, some as wives and mothers, and some will
turn out "not so good," thus bluntly summing up several decades of
Hollywood clichés about its female characters. The film's three subplots
are nested, in fact, in these three corresponding themes associated with
"the woman's film": sacrifice/stardom, marital crisis/renewal, and self-
destruction of the Fallen Woman. In the world according to *Ziegfeld
Girl*—a world established as "true" through decades of Ziegfeld publicity—these are the limits of female choices and female narratives.

As critics have noted with great interest, an additional level of "real-
life" stardom works in *Ziegfeld Girl* with the casting of actresses whose
performances and reputations call attention to themselves.[56] The casting
was also suggestive of Ziegfeld legends. Discovered-in-a-drugstore Lana
Turner melds smoothly into the generic discovered-by-Ziegfeld lore, and
Turner's brief, turbulent marriage in 1940 set her up as Sheila, a troubled,
vulnerable Lillian Lorraine type. Hedy Lamarr's exquisite exoticism and
mannequin coolness perfectly match her character Sandra, the ideal untouchable showgirl in the tradition of the *Follies'* most famous mannequin, Dolores; Judy Garland's earnest, stage-born, hardworking singer
and dancer Patty re-creates Ziegfeld's most talented women performers,
from Bessie McCoy through Marilyn Miller and Mary Eaton.

The foregrounding of these references—well-known performers por-
traying versions of other well-known performers—creates ironies and
dissonances that work against a coherent celebration of "Ziegfeldness"
or even a coherent meaning of the film's title. The tensions among
these ideals, references, and performances reach a crisis that literally
fragments the film, visually and in the plotline, during the grand finale
number, "You Gotta Pull Strings." This is the film's most Ziegfeldesque
extravaganza, featuring a song about Ziegfeld Girls that summarizes
decades of hype: "the newest crop of Mr. Z.'s girls," wearing "tons of
plumes and pearls," hailing from every state in the Union, and graduating from the "*Follies'* school . . . where beauty enters in the rough and
comes out labeled 'Glamour.' " Showcasing this product, "Glamour," the
staging glistens with legs and sparkly evening gowns, culminating in the
"Pretty Girl Is Like a Melody" tiered wedding cake–staircase footage

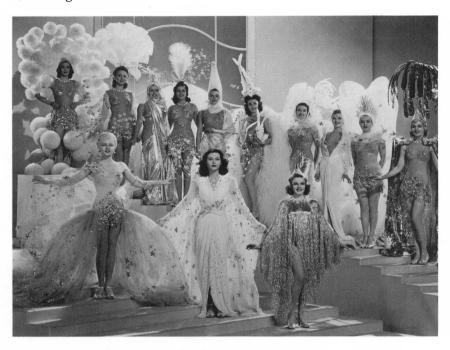

Lana Turner, Hedy Lamarr, and Judy Garland in revue costumes in *Ziegfeld Girl* (1941). (The Museum of Modern Art/Film Stills Archive)

lifted from *The Great Ziegfeld*, with an unlikely Judy Garland pasted into the top tier. The reverse shots for this number give us not the pleased spectator for whom this array is supposedly aimed but the miserable and dying Sheila, viewing the celebration of her former identity. The other out-of-place spectator is the Hedy Lamarr/Dolores–look-alike character, certainly the ideal trademark showgirl, who has renounced the *Follies* altogether and is watching from the balcony. The dislocations of spectacle/spectator (Judy Garland onstage as Glamour? Hedy Lamarr and Lana Turner in the audience?) signal the larger dislocation of the meaning of the Ziegfeld Girl of the title.

Perhaps the most tangled ambiguities accrue among Judy Garland, Lana Turner, their respective fictional characters, and the Ziegfeld star referents of these characters. Garland's physical appearance and star persona, even in regulation Ziegfeld costuming, works dismayingly against the trademark glamour, even though she is visually positioned as a top-of-the-tier Ziegfeld Girl.[57] In the final tiered-staircase number, she is wearing the same blond wig worn by the blond Audrey/Lillian Lorraine character who occupied this position in the 1936 film version of this number. The final shot tracks back from Garland's close-up and then fades into the original *Great Ziegfeld* footage, replacing her with the original Audrey/Lillian actress. Judy Garland doing Lillian Lorraine (via two other fictional characters, Audrey and Patty) is jarring enough, but this celebratory scene occurs as the other Lillian Lorraine reference, Sheila, is dying in the theater cloakroom, a Glorified American Girl who has succumbed to booze, sex, money, and other Fallen Woman temptations.

The visual, spatial, and referential fragmentations strongly suggest the sheer impossibility of locating and occupying that mythical position, the Ziegfeld Girl. A Ziegfeld Girl can be represented onstage ("Behold in us the newest crop of Mr. Ziegfeld's Girls," the women sing), but in the film's struggle to define a Ziegfeld Girl, the referent keeps slipping to other referents: "glamour" is Judy Garland as Patty as Audrey as Lillian Lorraine, but Lillian Lorraine is Lana Turner as Sheila, who is no longer even remotely glamorous and probably dead at the end of the narrative.

The impossibility of tracking down the Ziegfeld Girl is linked to the impossibility of tracking down Ziegfeld himself in this film, or even hearing his voice offstage, as occurs in later films. Instead, *Ziegfeld Girl* makes the showman an invisible, ubiquitous observer—on "voyages" of discovery on the streets of New York and in department store elevators—and the center of a wider surveillance system of managers and stage directors who test and filter out candidates for Ziegfeld Girls.[58] As the all-seeing god who must be pleased (Will Mr. Ziegfeld like the act? Will Mr. Ziegfeld approve the face, the figure, the song?) Ziegfeld operates as a code and discipline all the more powerful for its ability to be everywhere and nowhere. "Mr. Ziegfeld says if I don't watch my figure, no one else will," newly recruited Sheila explains to her mother about her new diet. The controlling gaze is no longer Ziegfeld's but is both internalized and deflected to the approving gazes of others.

The "Ziegfeld Girl" of the title refers, in this larger sense, to the impossible demands of bourgeois white femininity. The disembodied voice demanding the diet could be the voice of any 1920s (or 1941) fashion magazine advice column, urging both consumption and restraint, more luxuries, more pleasures, fewer calories, less flesh. Even the judgmental, selecting eye of Ziegfeld, ever watchful for raw beauty in department store elevators, only represents this larger cultural vision that privileges a specific body and face. The ideal creates unfillable gaps and insatiable desires: in short, the conditions of addiction, leading directly to Sheila's alcoholism and to her drunken fall from the stage platform, from the good graces of Ziegfeld, and from the code of respectable public female visibility.

The Ziegfeld Walk on the staircase, associated a number of times in this film with the Sheila character, summarizes the problems and contradictions of this wider social code.[59] Remember that the Walk was an artificial accommodation of body to architecture, a choreography of gender and class, and, by implication, a racialized choreography, a discipline of both the white "lady" and white fashion mannequin. Sources confirm that during the filming of Ziegfeld Girl, the story of "not-so-good" Sheila and the performance of Sheila by Lana Turner became more interesting to the filmmakers, who expanded the role so that it dominated the film. Discovered in a department store and confronted by Ziegfeld's advance man in a room full of display mannequins, Sheila is from the start invested in commodity culture and its assumptions about identity as a mode of wearing the body. Learning she will be a Ziegfeld Girl, her first response is to grab a fur coat from a saleswoman and order "three of these in different colors." Backstage, she quickly learns from a more experienced showgirl (Eve Arden) that a Ziegfeld Girl not only wears jewels and furs onstage but also can acquire them personally because she herself is valuable goods for exchange. Little wonder that the filmmakers became intrigued with Sheila's character and expanded her part to deal with its complexities—the complexities of being/having/losing the slippery identity of the consumable/consumer.

The class implications of the three Ziegfeld Girl plotlines suggest the relentless middlebrow appeal of Ziegfeld Girlhood, despite its upscale pretensions. The born-in-a-trunk Patty character is apparently immune to consumerist temptation because vaudeville has taught her to value talented performance over good looks; Patty eventually trades in her Peter Pan collars for fur ones, but she is not tempted to fashion-plate excesses. The classy Sandra is conveniently European, thus outside the embarrassments of commodified American class distinctions. Even in her showgirl performances, she exudes a quiet superiority to the revue business, rewarded eventually by her retirement to ladylike marriage with a Carnegie Hall artist. Only Sheila the elevator girl, daughter of an Irish Brooklyn cop, is vulnerable to the flashy baubles and trinkets of Ziegfeldness, a set of class desires and limitations that are specifically gendered. Without the work ethic of show business or the accustomed entitlements of class, Sheila enacts female versions of middlebrow success: upward mobility through looking and dressing a part and investment in the body as decor and (short-lived) pleasure for men.

The narrative didactically drives home the wrongheadedness of Sheila's superficiality and consumerist excesses. Sheila is owned by the trinkets and luxuries rather than vice versa. She is at the call of a man who sends limousine drivers looking for her; she trips and falls over her own fur coat. Unable to tell diamonds from glass, she eventually trades sexual favors for a gaudy dime-store brooch. Yet the production numbers of *Ziegfeld Girl* visually recuperate this excessiveness to the point of vulgarity, illustrating the slippage between Busby Berkeley's male-camera-eye choreography and the Marguerite Roberts–Sonya Levien screenplay, which seems to keep an eye on female conflicts and concerns. "You Stepped Out of a Dream" features the jewel-encrusted gowns, breathtaking hats, and lamé capes that are indeed the department store–elevator girl's dreams; "Minnie from Trinidad" enacts a gaudy tropical tourist brochure, with costumes that redesign women's bodies into exotic trees, bird's nests, and island foliage. And perhaps most problematical, one of the stagings of the grand finale number, "You Gotta Pull Strings," actually duplicates and multiplies Sheila's Fallen Woman penthouse boudoir, with twenty brass beds on which twenty showgirls toe-dance beneath silky canopies and a giant mirror. The song lyrics cynically advise (female) manipulation, instead of hard work, as the route to these riches: "If you want to go places, you want to see things, you gotta pull strings."

The film never resolves the relationship between these lush, desirable boudoir beddings and the ones in Sheila's sinful penthouse, but more explicitly than anything else in the film, they represent female sexuality itself, as a site constantly shifting among male desires, female spectacles, class values, and commodities. "Why can't the *men* you want have the *things* you want?" Sheila asks miserably at one point, trying to reconcile her love for a poor boyfriend and her love for furs and perfumes. When we do see female heterosexuality happily fulfilled, which occurs in the Sandra subplot, it takes place outside Ziegfeldness altogether, with former Ziegfeld Girl Sandra contentedly at her husband's side at the closure, both of them spectators of the elaborate show.

By 1941, the most obvious meaning of the Ziegfeld Girl was an upscale or respectable version of female sexual display for male pleasure. *Ziegfeld Girl* in fact opens with and often returns to a gallery scene of Glorified Girl portraits maintained by an adoring theater janitor. Yet this film powerfully demonstrates how that dynamic — female sexual imagery for a masculine gaze — was always more complicated in its actual implications and practices. American cultural and cinematic narratives could easily accommodate the story of Florenz Ziegfeld, artist of women's bodies, in Leonard's 1936 film. But when the focus turned to the famous Girl herself, the female fantasies she represented, and their class and social implications, Hollywood literally did not know what story to tell.

Beautiful White Bodies

The lavish Busby Berkeley numbers in *Ziegfeld Girl* insist on the spectatorial pleasures of showgirls, which the narrative scrambles to explain. Like the ornate costuming itself, the spectacles weigh down the film with their rich, troubling implications about gender, sexuality, fantasy, and riches. Furthering this argument about the Ziegfeld ideological legacy, I now turn to examples of Berkeley's earlier work, his staging and choreography in *Footlight Parade* and *Gold Diggers of 1933*, to track the social connotations of the visual production styles. My starting point is a singular visual effect that carries implications not immediately obvious: café au lait coloring and its evocation of the dusky belle.

The Ziegfeld Girl as dusky belle makes a subtle appearance in *Ziegfeld Girl*, when Judy Garland as Patty performs the specialty number "Minnie from Trinidad." This is one of the film's tributes to original *Follies* numbers, in this case the song "Miss Ginger of Jamaica," from the *Fol-*

lies' 1907 premier. While the original song had emphasized the singer's racial exoticism, "doing things up brown," as the lyrics proclaim, the song Garland delivers about islander Minnie is a bleached, Disney-style ballad that justifies onstage donkeys, straw hats, and palm trees, one of which sprouts from Garland's head. "Minnie," after all, is a comic number; at one point, Garland sings to the donkey, who also wears a funny straw hat.

Garland's makeup is a light café au lait, perhaps approximating the color of people in Ziegfeldian Trinidad, but it also approximates Garland's makeup in another 1941 performance, the minstrel number "Waiting for the Robert E. Lee" in *Babes on Broadway*, directed and choreographed by Busby Berkeley. In this number, Garland's feminine blackface is several shades lighter than the grotesque version worn by her partner, Mickey Rooney. On one level, Garland's two high-yellow performances reference each other as reminders of her theatrical virtuosity; blackface was a staple of the theatrical tradition that is the theme of both films. But on another level, considering the function of blackface as masquerade and as acknowledgment of racial difference, these performances also reinforce Garland's own ambiguous star status as "different," not glamorous, not quite in sync with Hollywood's categories of attractive heterosexuality.[60] Garland's on-screen blackface premier had actually occurred in the 1939 *Babes in Arms'* minstrel number (also directed and choreographed by Berkeley) in which she and Rooney both wear traditional dark blackface with exaggerated white mouths. As Minnie and as the minstrel miss on Rooney's arm, Garland represents her own paradoxical marginality as an MGM star, a factor that aligns her with the camp readings of Ziegfeld that I discuss in the epilogue of this book.

In short, the Minnie performance and the similar café au lait performance in *Babes on Broadway* that same year foreground Garland's status as not-exactly-Ziegfeld Girl, significantly registered here in both racial and sexual terms. The "not-exactly-Ziegfeld" status is the gap between the overt sexuality of the original "Ginger from Jamaica" and its comic version as "Minnie." As opposed to the sexy, bad-girl, dusky belle performances occasionally taken on by Ziegfeld Girls, Ziegfeld's women coon shouters were comics: Fanny Brice, Sophie Tucker, Nora Bayes. Their variety acts punctuated the grand Girl displays; they were the defining, contrasting "bodies between" the displays of Glorified Girls, like the dancer in the other costume color witnessed by Edmund Wilson. The effect of a suntanned Judy Garland in "Minnie" is similar; the real Ziegfeld Girls, the Lana Turner and Hedy Lamarr characters, float or pose in the same number, in no way connected with the comedy of the donkeys and the plump, decidedly nonromantic Don Pedro to whom Garland sings.

During the Ziegfeld era, the dusky belle of white revues was both a reference to and a displacement of her black counterpart in the *Darktown Follies* and in the black musicals. Similarly, Garland's blackface in MGM musicals exemplifies the loss and absence of black female talent on-screen in those musical films after *Hallelujah* (1929).[61] The elaborate *Babes on Broadway* minstrel number, with its surprising reversals of white costumes and black faces, suggests a photographic negative, but the reversals actually go the other way: white bodies have replaced the black ones from the lively tradition of black musicals that would not have much of a cinematic life. Berkeley's choreography was infused with black-white patterning as visual design that, in the minstrel numbers in *Babes in Arms* and *Babes on Broadway,* cleverly enacts the black-white tensions of musical theater.[62] These moments relentlessly delineate color lines by invoking and representing what has been banished, just as the black chorus girl was both forbidden but vividly pantomimed on the Ziegfeld stage to specify the whiteness of the Glorified Girl.

A similar dynamic of substitution and racial definition can be glimpsed in the uses of Berkeley's chorus girls in *Footlight Parade* (1933). This film contains no blackface, but in its most telling moment of dislocation and disavowal, it reimagines African American children as white showgirls. Preoccupied about ideas for his new production number, the harried director character played by James Cagney looks off-camera, in a well-lit medium shot on a busy street, at the sound of water and voices. "Look at that!" he exclaims with the excited earnestness that is the backstage musical's code for inspiration. "That's what that prologue needs! A mountain waterfall splashing on beautiful white bodies!"

The eyeline match shot, however, is not a waterfall and "beautiful white bodies" but rather a grainy, dimly lit long shot of a black neighborhood; African American children play around a gushing fire hydrant, while in the background, blurred sidewalk figures of a black crowd look on. In the plotline, the ensuing stage production inspired by this scene is one of Busby Berkeley's most baroque numbers, "By a Waterfall," in which hundreds of Anglo female bodies swim, twirl, glide, and cavort supposedly as part of an elaborate theatrical prologue, though filmed and edited as a physically impossible fantasy.

The other physically impossible fantasy, an African American scene transformed into an upscale white production, involves a more basic but ideologically powerful visual trick. The Cagney character, Chester Kent, literally cannot see blackness except as a way of seeing whiteness.[63] The edited sequence offers the same "white" reading to the viewer: a medium shot of Cagney exclaiming about "beautiful white bodies" is followed by the eyeline match of what he sees, the grainy shot of the black children in the black neighborhood. The darkness and distance of the countershot ensure that the black faces are not clearly visible. Berkeley's "By a Waterfall" acts out the preferred, white, upscale alternative to darker bodies in another, less valuable scene.

In the following shot, Cagney excitedly asks an attending policeman, "Do you get it?" The policeman, caught up in the enthusiasm of Cagney's inspiration, suddenly becomes a show business entrepreneur himself. "I have ideas too, Mr. Kent!" he exclaims as he jumps into Cagney's car, which takes them both to the theater. The double prompting of the producer and the street cop implies an interplay of pleasure and policing—entertainment and constraint—that is rarely suggested so blatantly in Hollywood cinema. Racial visibility in 1930s cinema had been addressed by a ban on the representation of miscegenation in the Production Code, the film industry's self-censorship apparatus, which was adopted in 1930 and enforced rigorously after 1933. But interracial relationships in Hollywood studio films were also thoroughly prohibited on the level of narrative spectatorship and performance. A light-skinned black performer such as Nina Mae McKinney could perform within an all-black cast of *Hallelujah*, but a cinematic taboo hovered around the scenario of a sexually provocative black performance for a white audience—the dynamics of Harlem nightclubs or previous black musicals—as if this spectator relationship alone suggested miscegenation.[64] Generally, this cinematic coding and taboo keep invisible the racial dimensions of sexual

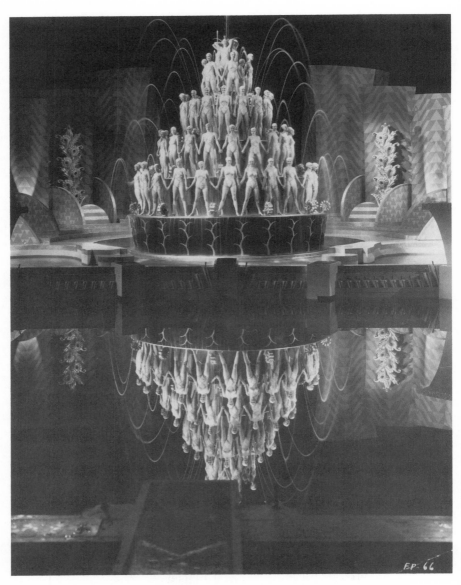

"By a Waterfall," choreographed by Busby Berkeley, in *Footlight Parade* (1933).
(The Museum of Modern Art/Film Stills Archive)

desire. The cop in *Footlight Parade*, as a representative of legal power and its supposedly comic complicity in this scene — "I have ideas too" — is particularly ominous in light of the fact that the resulting "By a Waterfall" sequence was, Mast tells us, "a great favorite of Adolf Hitler."[65]

The Cagney character, Chester Kent, was probably based on Chester Hale, musical prologue producer of New York's Capitol Theater (c. 1925–38), who, along with Ziegfeld, utilized the choreography of Ned Wayburn. Prologue choreographers were expected to create new shows weekly, which often toured large theaters that could accommodate fairly extravagant productions.[66] Kent, who is characterized as a quick-minded, endlessly energetic perfectionist in charge of hundreds of showgirls, also more than slightly resembles the public persona of Ziegfeld himself, the "manager of unfailing resource . . . a trim, athletic, fastidiously groomed young man" who "keeps his alertly inventive mind working like a machine gun." Ziegfeld had died just two years before this film was made, and *Footlight Parade* can easily be read as one of his posthumous Hollywood beatifications.

Like Ziegfeld watching his best stars go to Hollywood, Chester early in this film watches dejectedly as crowds throng the new talking-picture theater, abandoning the musical theater of Broadway. Chester resolves this problem through two highly inventive inspirations during the course of the plotline. The black street scene gives him the idea for a stunning novelty number. Earlier, he is inspired when he buys cheap, mass-produced aspirin and suddenly realizes that he can mass-produce musical prologues. The first inspiration takes place in a drugstore, the second on a city street, locations clearly outside the theaters where Chester works. But Chester repeatedly shows that for him there is no outside to this theater, as evidenced in his "seeing" the street scene as a musical revue. As theorists of the musical genre have pointed out, this approach to "the world as entertainment" is a common cue for a character's heroism or likability; in the backstage musical in particular, it reinforces the sense of the show business world as microcosm or more intense version of the world outside the theater.[67]

In *Footlight Parade* this theatrical "world" represents not just entertainment but a classed and racialized economy as well. As more recent film history has emphasized, the sumptuous movie palaces of the type portrayed in *Footlight Parade*—theaters large enough to stage musical productions—were showcases themselves, offering class-specific ideas about fashion, leisure, and decor: chandeliers, thick carpeting, velvet drapes. So the theater itself demarcated no clear boundary between the opulence of the stage productions and the opulence of the architecture or between desirable accoutrements inside the theater and those outside. In *Footlight Parade*, there is not even a clear demarcation between the glamour of the diegetic theater audience and the glamour onstage. The men in these audiences wear tuxedos, and the women wear fashionable gowns that match, in upscale fashion, the costuming they are seeing in the stage productions. This mirroring effect represses the status of the "work" onstage by suggesting a continuum of a privileged world of leisure and visual pleasure. The audience that has purchased this view and this fantasy sees itself idealized in a display in which working-class young women masquerade as elegantly attired showgirls. When the three grand revue numbers, including "By a Waterfall," erupt out of any logical narrative space, the dissolution of boundary is complete.[68]

This presents a dilemma, for commodity value cannot be established without hierarchical differences. In the "By a Waterfall" number, the effect of the identical white bodies performing for the identically white audience requires another location, an "outside," a site of lesser value. The space of the movie palace can be valuable only if some other site is not. The glimpse of the black neighborhood underscores what might otherwise be taken for granted: that the glamour of the movie palace depends on its racial whiteness. As Richard Dyer argues in a 1988 essay, whiteness as a "norm" needs to be constructed, paradoxically because whiteness is "everything and nothing," which is precisely "the source of its representational power." An effective strategy of construction, Dyer suggests, is "reference to that which is not white, as if only non-whiteness can give whiteness any substance."[69] The reference to the black children in the "Waterfall" performance operates as such a construction, handily doubling the sexual value of the showgirls as a conflated economic and racial desirability.

Racial difference signifies sexual desirability here, but desirability cannot even be divisible into racial, sexual, and economic registers in this film. The "beautiful white bodies" are powerful because they are not reducible to any one of these registers without the implication of the others. Within a narrative saturated with anxieties about business, money, and profits, certain showgirl bodies have economic value only within a particular theater, which in turn must occupy a hierarchical space. The shot of the black children in the street provides a glimpse of another theater, so to speak, a black neighborhood in which children play and curious spectators line the sidewalk. A number of devaluations occur with this shot. Most obvious, as a "depression musical," *Footlight Parade* relegates poverty—which affected blacks and whites alike—to blackness, literalized as the impoverished production values in this dim, fuzzy shot of the black neighborhood. When this scene is transformed, whitened, and reenacted as the "Waterfall" number within the movie palace, the desirability of the showgirls has been located within many other social desires. Within the movie palace, displays of the jewelry, satins, tuxedos, chandeliers, velvet curtains, and showgirls—that is, the visual displays on both sides of the stage—have value and meaning because of what has been glimpsed and excluded.

The anxious contention about entertainment value—a "real" Broadway as opposed to a black entertainment scene—has very discernible sources in New York City nightlife during this era, as I described in the last chapter. When *Footlight Parade* was made in the early 1930s, the clubs of Harlem were still providing a thriving black musical scene that for white audiences was thrilling and transgressive. From 1925 to 1935, white customers flocked to these clubs looking for enactments of white fantasies about black sensuality and "primitive" black sexiness, especially as embodied in lighter-skinned black women. These Harlem performers, like the chorus girls in the African American revues, provided a racial/sexual alternative to the middle-class "niceness" of the Ziegfeld Girl. The denial made by Chester Kent on the street, seeing beautiful white bodies instead of black children, is very much a denial of the threatening uptown scene with its alluring black showgirls. The Ziegfeld history provides one of the frameworks by which this racial construction would have made cultural sense as a 1930s text: the Glorified American Girl performs at the New Amsterdam or Ziegfeld Theater, while darker women "glorifying the Creole beauty" dance in a less expensive musical on another street.

My argument here has been that Berkeley's women as mass-produced images materialize and complete the production of women as glorified and trademarked, "an actual process invented by Zieggy." One of my larger arguments in this book is that the Ziegfeld Girl's two most obvious trademark features, her whiteness and her heterosexuality, were contended sites of definition during the Ziegfeld era. Whereas *Footlight Parade* suggests the racial significance of the showgirl body, Mervyn LeRoy's *Gold Diggers of 1933*, also choreographed by Berkeley, foregrounds the importance and slippery marketability of her heterosexuality. Like the black street scene glimpsed in *Footlight Parade*, the two "other scenes" glimpsed and recuperated in *Gold Diggers* are prostitution and, less obviously, lesbianism. Prostitution is hardly a subtle subtext in a film about gold digging, but the film's cynicism about this issue—Ginger Rogers and the chorus girls wear giant gold coins in the opening production number—implies that for women, desire is no prerequisite for sexual relationships with men.

The relatively long cultural life of Avery Hopwood's 1919 play *Gold Diggers* attests to the popularity of this snappy, comic chorus girl story. *Gold Diggers* ran for two years on Broadway with former Ziegfeld Girl Ina Claire as its star and then went on tour. Warner Brothers produced a silent film version in 1923 and a musical version, *Gold Diggers of Broadway*, in 1929. The latter was so successful that the Warners remade the film in 1933, 1935, and 1936; the story resurfaced once more on Broadway Television Theater in 1952. In every version, a romantic plotline of mistaken identities and backstage shenanigans eventually matches chorus girls to wealthy men, a narrative no doubt made credible by real-life chorines who had made careers out of such associations—including Ziegfeld Girls Marion Davies and Peggy Hopkins Joyce.[70]

The 1933 film version of *Gold Diggers* foregrounds issues of money and employment by specifically citing the depression and its impact on theater, in the narrative itself and in its best-known production numbers, "In the Money" and "Remember My Forgotten Man," the latter a tribute to unemployed World War I veterans. The presence of a sympathetic prostitute in "Forgotten Man" is a clue about the film's theme, for the narrative and staging of *The Gold Diggers of 1933* suggest straightforwardly that the only reliable work for women is sex—illegally, as prostitution, or legally, as marriage. Gold digging, conveniently enough, refers to both.

Berkeley's chorus girl numbers in this film amplify previous, accumulated meanings of the chorus girl's body as a product suitable for show. Campy and outright kinky at times, the chorines appear as sparkling currency or "canned goods" to be pried open for pleasure ("Pettin' in the Park"). Not surprisingly, the chorus girl body as prized commodity is given distinctively Ziegfeldian connotations through the costumes, sets, and choreography. The elaborate stagings involve staircases, creative lighting effects, and platforms; the costuming and choreography are matched to the elaborate sets, so that the floral pattern in the staging of "The Shadow Waltz" rhymes with petal-shaped skirts.[71] The Ziegfeldian lavishness is a strong marker of predepression plenitude, reinforcing what film historians call the utopian dimension of the musical. *Gold Diggers of 1933*, however, harshly contrasts these utopian theatrical numbers with the grim economic realities of theatrical workers, the chorines who do not get paid when the show closes down.

As most of the film's critics point out, women's work and the necessity of working for a living are foregrounded in this film. The chorus girls are represented as independent, often sassy, resourceful modern women. Yet the film is unable to represent any woman's paid work except onstage. One hard-up chorus girl claims to be working in a drugstore, but she is never seen there, so the only work visualized for women is the chorus line. The most forward gold digger of them all, played by Ginger Rogers, is explicitly marked as sexually active; one of her colleagues cracks that the male show producer would not know her "with clothes on." The film goes to great pains to expose the contradictions in the women's economic predicaments and in men's foolishness in falling for superficial female images. The priggish, wealthy characters J. Lawrence and Peabody dismiss the vulgarity of theater women but are also drawn to them—and in the spirit of good, satirical romantic comedy, they eventually marry them, though this will also transform the chorines into respectable society wives. The dynamic is familiar from Ziegfeld advertising and hype: upscale setting and costume creates, for women, a direct visual relationship with an upper class and enables her class mobility. The access is possible because she has been choreographed into behavior that fits the visual package: the beaded evening gown and the elbow-length gloves are the wearing of a discipline. At their most Ziegfeldian, the chorus girls in this film form a giant neon violin, a reference to classical music and its milieu, to which they have access literally through their bodies as plastic, malleable elements in a larger design.

Gold Diggers of 1933 has attracted a great deal of critical attention, especially by feminist film theorists, because its excessive spectacles, outrageous production numbers, and female ensemble cast offer rich, multiple, often contradictory readings. The startling first musical number alone, in which commodified chorus girls are literalized as currency, doppled with gold coins from hair to crotch, has been described as camp comedy, depression-era cynicism, unabashed voyeurism, Foucauldian power paradigms, sexual and commodity fetishism, and spoofs of anti-prostitution reform discourse.[72] That is, the woman-as-currency visual metaphor immediately brings to bear both historical and psychoanalytic frameworks, as well as readings that tend to veer in extreme directions, from misogyny to feminist camp.

The Ziegfeld history, as an additional context for this film, sheds light on the ambiguities of the showgirl figure herself, given the Ziegfeldian agenda to elevate the chorus girl to a "pricey item" and downplay her connotations as prostitute and contemptible property—all of which are registered in the course of the 1933 *Gold Diggers*. Yet *Gold Diggers* also reveals how heterosexuality—the linchpin of the entire chorine economy—can be comprised of purchasing power and "work" rather than desire. The upscale showgirl, Berkeley's version of the Ziegfeld Girl as gold coin or violin in this film, is commodified and publicized as heterosexual because the economy supports it, not because there is an innate physical or psychological inclination, or even a pleasure, involved from her perspective. Pamela Robertson's reading of this film, emphasizing its appeal to female spectators, argues its stark social message about women's lack of choices in a depressed economy and in a visual/mass-media economy as well, so that prostitution or self-commodification becomes a necessity for survival.[73] I would add that heterosexuality itself is necessary for survival in *Gold Diggers*—or at least the appearance and maintenance of heterosexuality, which is the more important question pushed by the excessive Ziegfeldian performances of the "model" woman/commodity/mannequin/showcase Girl. This is the case because desire, even more than whiteness, is impossible to "see" and thus must be explicitly choreographed. Its choreography becomes more apparent,

however, with slippages of difference, just as the whiteness of the Ziegfeld Girl is made more apparent by the inclusion of Minnie from Trinidad, Ginger of Jamaica, and café au lait.

By questioning the status and locations of female desire, prostitutes
and lesbians have always been culturally linked as figures threatening the
organization of heterosexuality. The chorus girl is part of this grouping
because as a working girl she disengages or denaturalizes female dependence on men, reframing that dependence as a business exchange. *Gold
Diggers of 1933* exemplifies these issues of female public visibility and self-
commodification that had always hovered around the chorus girl figure.
Frothy media representations of the chorus girl marked an underlying
excitement and trepidation about a more serious, if displaced image:
a line of women on the job, women who work in the public sphere.
As pointed out in Chapter 2, the chorus girl as a figure of modernity
was split between cutting-edge and retrograde discourses: on one hand,
the new female independence in mixed-sex working and leisure worlds
and, on the other hand, the connotations of the oldest profession in
the world, a continuation of traditional negative connotations about
actresses.[74] Just as more women entered and stayed in the workforce,
slowly moving into professional fields, the chorus girl role suggested
that women's continuing work is sex, an extension of the private realm,
thus also reinforcing the notion that women's "real" work is making
themselves presentable for show.

In *Gold Diggers of 1933*, the comic character Trixie (Aline MacMahon)
provides a slippage of difference, unsettling some of the cultural assumptions about this sexual work. Trixie, the oldest and toughest of
the three chorine heroines, is never neatly aligned into a coherent sex-
gender visual sign and is the character who most blatantly discusses
heterosexuality as a business. Within the codes of the film, the actress
Aline MacMahon is the least conventionally attractive of the costars, her
long features and large body a clear contrast to the standardized cuteness and smallness of Ruby Keeler, Joan Blondell, and Ginger Roberts.
For Trixie, marriage is an alternative occupation not necessarily connected to love or romance: "When show business was slow, I used to
live on my alimony. Now I can't collect a cent of it. Married three of
them against a rainy day. Now it's pouring and they haven't an umbrella

between them!"[75] Hard times and Trixie's scheming lead to yet a fourth marriage, to the elderly Peabody, another exchange of sex for financial security, with minimal sentimental touches.

The ambiguity of Trixie, the not-quite-glamorous version of the chorus girl, is also apparent in Hank in *Broadway Melody* and Patty in *Ziegfeld Girl,* recurring characters who resist the "safer" meanings of the chorus girl as pleasure for men/exhibitionist desire of women. As opposed to the romantic comedy enacted by the other chorus girls in this film, Trixie's comedy is bawdy and less feminine—the comedy of camp, as Robertson points out, and also the comedy of the "unruly woman," smart-mouthed and aggressive.[76]

Trixie's comedy also undercuts the more glamorous enactments of gold digging in the production numbers (the association with glittery costumes and gorgeous women) and in the plotline's romanticism (the "true" love of J. Lawrence and chorine Carol). In addition, her comedy undermines the heterosexuality of these couplings, in which female sexuality may only be a convenient arrangement. In the exchange of sexuality and gold, there is always an ambiguity about who has been cheated and who has been exploited, an ambiguity of the "value" of sexual pleasure and desire.[77] In the chorus girl–gold digger paradigm, female pleasure is usually associated with the jewelry, hats, and general financial security sought by the women characters. Two of the subplots code this transaction as romance, but the Trixie character employs a different code altogether.

Mellencamp notes that Trixie is "cross-dressed as a policewoman" in the kinky "Pettin' in the Park" number.[78] The oddness of this description (how can a woman be cross-dressed as a woman?) belies its accuracy. In this dance number, Trixie is shot three-quarter length in her uniform coat and cap, so the effect is definitely drag. Trixie's cop is a joke, with a number of male policemen/dancers reminding us that this is men's work and that women doing such work are transgressive. Cross-dressed, MacMahon as Trixie could easily be an inscription of the mannish and possibly lesbian career woman, the embodiment of the "unnatural" place of woman in the workforce. She reappears in this costume, strangely enough, in the penultimate scene revealing the three united couples, when she announces that she is a bride, and the incongruous effect underscores the humor of her character. Again, the effect is drag until the next shot reframes her and reveals that along with the cap and uniform top, she is actually wearing a skirt.

The comedy of this costume for Trixie slyly insists on its sexual twist. The comic cops in "Pettin' in the Park" are policing sexual activity, acting as bourgeois (and hence laughable) social constraints on natural activity, male-female coupling. So Trixie is doubly out of place, as an outsider to the heterosexuality on display and as a transgressive female body in the customary place of a man. There is nothing cutesy about Trixie in drag—this is not Ginger Rogers in a sailor suit but Alice MacMahon looking butch and confirming the nonalignment of Trixie's character with the romantic trappings that make gold digging acceptable. My emphasis here on the sexual instability of Trixie's character and plotline only continues what the film already posits as funny: that gold digging creates strange bedfellows. The Trixie-Peabody arrangement is especially incongruous in its mismatches of ages, classes, and personalities, but Trixie's semiotic mismatches scramble the sexual pairing here as well.

Just a year before the release of this film, a less cynical version of chorines rising to wealth appeared in *Blondie of the Follies* (1932), which starred two former Ziegfeld Girls, Marion Davies and Billie Dove. Its advertisements in Hearst newspapers made the biographical connection of Blondie and Marion Davies unmistakable: "Blondie's amazing career, from tenement obscurity to the dazzling heights of Broadway fame, is a story so interesting we can no longer keep it from you. Thrilling romance . . . popular acclaim . . . parties . . . penthouse apartment . . . all part of her soul-stirring struggle for success."[79] The plotline of this film, positing the big break for two chorus girls through their associations with wealthy men, indeed sketches out Davies's "amazing career." In the familiar wife-or-showgirl dichotomy, one showgirl chooses marriage, the other a show business career, in the comforting *Broadway Melody* tradition.

Marion Davies's rise from chorus girl to Ziegfeld Girl to film star provided a titillating, real-life narrative for this era. William Randolph Hearst was captivated by Davies's performance in a 1915 Broadway revue. By the time she was "glorified" by Ziegfeld in the *Follies* the next year, she was Hearst's mistress, shamelessly publicized in his newspapers as an outstanding showgirl. Her biographer, Fred Lawrence Guiles, claims the journalistic promotions suggested her role in the *Follies* was far greater than it actually was; even though she is frequently cited as "ex-Ziegfeld Girl," her career with Ziegfeld lasted no more than a year—a clue to the *Follies'* prestige. The caption over her full-page photo in a 1916 *American Weekly* read "Marion Davies, the Type of Chorus Girl Who Marries Captains of Industry and Coronets: For Every Man, There's 'One Dangerous Girl.' "[80] Hearst did not marry his "dangerous girl," but his publicity helped launch her from the *Follies* to other stage work and eventually to Hollywood, where she would star in Hearst's film company. While *Blondie of the Follies* has fairly disappeared from cultural memory, Davies's far more enduring cinematic presence is her metonymic appearance as the hysterical Susan Alexander in *Citizen Kane*, a representation that unfortunately elides Davies's considerable comic talent in her own film work.

Blondie and Susan Alexander suggest respectively the frothy fairy tale and the bitter melodramatic versions of the woman staged by an ambitious man. Likewise, the Cinderella version of the Ziegfeld Girl (*Sally*) competes with its darker rendition (Lana Turner in *Ziegfeld Girl*) in cinema because her meanings have always hovered between reversible cultural images of women: consumer/consumable, working girl/gold digger, chorus girl/call girl. Even the golden Gloria of *Glorifying the American Girl* suffers in her swift trajectory from department store to *Follies* display, learning only in the finale that she has exchanged womanhood for an iconic abstraction—icy mannequin perfection. Ziegfeld's favorite, stuffy, pretentious word for it was "pulchritude," with which the Ziegfeld Girl in film was both blessed and afflicted.

EPILOGUE

Showgirls

Showgirls are still with us. In the 1990s, several generations after Ziegfeld claimed he invented them, showgirls have appeared in a *New Yorker* photo portfolio by Annie Leibovitz, in the eponymous major film by Paul Verhoeven, and in Las Vegas casino shows called *Jubilee!* and *Enter the Night*. A recent *New York Times Magazine* essay points out that as Las Vegas turns into a theme park, showgirls now compete with water slides as tourist attractions, although they remain a reliable niche of "old fashioned smut."[1]

Their great-grandmother, the Ziegfeld Girl, while not directly referenced in these shows and texts, is still with us as well, a residual image that apparently retains some punch. A 1996 *New Yorker* essay by John Lahr titled "My Mother the Ziegfeld Girl" asks as its header question, "What was a Ziegfeld Girl about?" She was about glamour, according to her son, who remembers his mother well into senior citizenship still able to pull off the haughty smile ("a sense of aloofness and decorum") and even the Walk, giving the impression of being "at once unattainable and irresistible."[2]

Many years ago, a former Ziegfeld Girl lived downstairs from me in an old stone mansion subdivided into charming and haunted apartments. She was Lina Basquette, star of Cecil B. DeMille's *Godless Girl*, dancer and celebrity of stage and screen. In 1989, an in-depth *New Yorker* piece on Basquette detailed her meteoric career and savory private life.[3] But in the previous decade, Basquette was mostly a good-natured source for occasional feature stories in the local newspaper, where she was usually introduced not as star of the 1929 DeMille film but as "former Ziegfeld Girl." Still an elegant figure well into her seventies, she would walk imperiously through the terraced gardens overlooking the town, and I would peer through my screened kitchen window, smitten voyeur of the godless showgirl.

From that distance, Basquette too was unattainable and irresistible. Friends and interviewers found her otherwise, and her anecdotes and gossip were legendary for their snap and bite. Of her boxes of written memoirs, several hundred pages went into print as an autobiography crammed with scandalous recollections, culminating with her (often repeated) tour de force, the night Adolf Hitler attempted to seduce her: "Come, Liebchen, kiss the pain away. Beg forgiveness from your Führer —" "Please, Adolf, I beg you. Think about EVA!" [4] As this suggests, the B-movie dialogue that fills her book does not hold up as well as my memories, in which she haughtily presides over terrace and town.

Ziegfeld's investment in his Girl very much depended on the controlled distance and aura of The Genuine Article, utterly removed from mortal touch, self-published star biographies, or B movies. Likewise, John Lahr's affectionate memoir portrays a woman whose sense of Ziegfeld Girl allure far outlasted the age of mechanical reproduction. Just six months before Lahr's article appeared, Leibovitz's photo portfolio in the same magazine included contemporary Las Vegas showgirls, topless, in full Ziegfeldesque glory: spangled headdresses, elbow-length gloves, wreaths of jewels above and between their breasts. In a 1920s Ziegfeld revue, the seminudity would have been dramatized and occluded by low lighting and transparent curtains, a costly sight only for well-dressed ticket holders at the New Amsterdam Theater. In the *New Yorker*, the photographs have dramatic value as statements about the material construction of glamour, for Leibovitz also included black and white photo portraits of the showgirls in their street clothes, without makeup, in eyeglasses, one with her children. The stunning effect of the portfolio is not the seminudity but the utter ordinariness of the women previous to their transformation by glue-on eyelashes, net stockings, Kodachrome, and beads. The showgirls photographed by Leibovitz are students and mothers who dress up because the pay is good and the work is steady, with no illusions about stardom, discovery, and rising from the chorus.

The Leibovitz showgirls are most of all reproducible, by a best-selling weekly magazine and by the tricks of eyeliner and a good lens. The uniqueness of the Ziegfeld Girl, her maddening unattainability, depended on mystification (she was glorified!) and exclusive physical presence. Even within the Ziegfeld enterprise, the chorines chosen by various musical directors for the road shows were not considered "real"

Ziegfeld Girls, the ones hand-selected by Ziegfeld himself. More than that, mass reproduction—of celebrity, cable channels, videos, pornography, Demi Moore's body in a movie about strippers—has produced female sexuality as both knowable and multiple in its meanings. The Las Vegas showgirl on the staircase with her teasing feathers no longer tests a limit of female visibility or suggests the facts of life, as Anna Held presumably did for the turn-of-the-century bride. Even the latent sexualities of the showgirl have been explicitly illustrated by Madonna in her book and videos; a lesbian characterization in Verhoeven's 1996 *Showgirls* was panned by critics as both phony and clichéd.

Given these demystifications, the question is why a Ziegfeldesque showgirl appears at all in the last decade of the twentieth century, with or without the explicit trademark reference, as the bejeweled *New Yorker* portrait, the Las Vegas attraction, or as herself, a character in Broadway shows such as *The Will Rogers Follies* and *Ziegfeld: A Night at the Follies*. Certainly part of her long-term appeal is the mixed corniness and eroticism of her previously shocking history. The generic Las Vegas showgirl, associated with glitz, luck, and neon, points backward, to a time when the acknowledgment of sex as currency was still transgressively brazen. At the beginning of this century, the fictional showgirl in McCardell's novel *Conversations of a Chorus Girl* confides with mock naïveté, "I'm from one of the best families of Altoona, Pa., and my mother would die if she knew I wore tights on the road." Her sexual meaning as valuable goods was still an open secret. Today's showgirls, like the Berkeley chorines costumed as giant coins in *Gold Diggers of 1933,* are so obvious as to be either embarrassing or kitsch. Creatures of spandex and sequins, showgirls like the ones glimpsed in the Martin Scorsese film *Casino* (1996) are predictable and brightly colored background sights that "prove" Las Vegas is thrilling and provocative. The status of the showgirl as tourist attraction for busloads of California suburbanites or planeloads of vacationers from the East ensures her artificial shock value.

The Ziegfeld Girl herself is likewise a regressive figure, still recognizable as a bundle of signs associated with a glamorous past. Her value is often sentimental as much as kitschy, the sentiment very much romanticizing a supposedly more innocent era of commodification. Despite the Ziegfeld enterprise's horrified distance from vamps and flappers, the Jazz Age and the Ziegfeld Girl have become conflated as early models of sexiness and conspicuous consumption. The Glorified Girls of the two aforementioned Broadway shows are outfitted with an abundance of feather boas and specifically linked to this era of the *Follies*. The Ziegfeld extravaganzas in these shows are symbols and celebrations of pre-1929 excessiveness. "It's 1927, and every girl dreams of being a Ziegfeld Girl," one character announces early in *A Night at the Follies*. The dreamiest and most imaginative element in this play is costuming; the show's publicity emphasized that over four hundred thousand beads and feathers were used for the three hundred costumes seen onstage, many of which evoked more applause than the players. In *The Will Rogers Follies*, the lavish *Follies* showgirl display appears dramatically the moment before the 1929 crash itself, which is represented as the defrocking of the Glorified Girls.

The nostalgia for the costumes and glittery spectacle of Ziegfeld is nostalgia for the Girl as well. The plotline of *A Night at the Follies*, of three would-be Glorified Girls and their romances, virtually retells the 1941 *Ziegfeld Girl* film, but as a fluffy comedy, with no melodramatic overtones. The plot's conflicts—marriage or the stage? domesticity or stardom?—fantasize and simplify dilemmas about working women and women's "place," imagining a fun-filled 1920s when those issues were quickly resolvable. Expensive frivolity was the whole point of the *Follies* era and Girl, the play insists. Likewise, the showgirls in *The Will Rogers Follies* are associated with a golden era characterized by Will Rogers himself. The substitution of Rogers (monogamy, folk wisdom, cowboy simplicity) for Ziegfeld (excessive spending, womanizing, and whim) sanitizes and bowdlerizes the *Follies* into a kinder, gentler enterprise. In turn, the rise-to-stardom narrative focuses on Rogers rather than one of the showgirls, eliminating muddy issues of celebrity and illusion. Rogers, we are told in this play, was always simply himself. (This claim could hardly hold with Eddie Cantor, Bert Williams, and Bert Savoy, the other well-known male Ziegfeld stars, famous respectively for white blackface, black blackface, and female impersonation.) As a result, the showgirls in *The Will Rogers Follies* symbolize Ziegfeld's trademark glamour and Rogers's historical milieu as part of the nostalgia package, marker of an era when men, women, and feather boas were obviously what they were.

The representations of Ziegfeld in these plays continue the omnipotence tradition beginning with the films *Ziegfeld Girl* and *Ziegfeld Follies* in the 1940s, in which Ziegfeld is either the offstage presence or the minor god in a heaven/balcony. In *Will Rogers*, Ziegfeld is the resonant voice of Gregory Peck emitted from the back of the theater, all-powerful but unseen. In *A Night at the Follies*, he is represented only by the back of a coated figure, a mannequin rolled out between the audience and the stage at key moments. The dynamic is not just voyeuristic but also panoptic, as I have suggested in previous chapters, situating an invisible surveillance of appearance and behavior. In *The Will Rogers Follies*, the leggy, scantily clad showgirl discreetly named Ziegfeld's favorite sashays occasionally onstage, ever mindful of her Big Daddy in the wings, to deliver messages to Will. In the New York production, she was played for a while by Marla Maples, the woman who would be Donald Trump's, a casting triumph that caps the Ziegfeld Girl's meanings as class marker and ornament, golden and gold digger, pulchritude and prize.

The female body as commercial trademark or guarantee continues to have explicitly racial implications in mainstream advertising and in practices ranging from pornography to Las Vegas showgirl routines. A good example is Verhoeven's *Showgirls* film, which salaciously flaunted onscreen sexual taboos but avoided the racial-sexual ones; showgirls represented in this version of ribald sexuality and Las Vegas are without exception white.

The "aesthetic" policy of the Rockettes, requiring white showgirls, prevailed until 1987, when the hiring of a single black woman sent management and dance direction into chaos. Patricia J. Williams reads this as an example of the failure of tokenism; to make different-colored chorus girls work aesthetically, she points out, you need to include a number of darker-skinned women who could in fact create color patterns with their lighter-skinned colleagues. For that matter, she asks, why not also hire a variety of skin shades, including lighter-skinned black women like the ones from Cotton Club days?[5] This question cuts to the very heart of a pop culture institution such as the Rockettes and its identity as *not* the Cotton Club—as a "better," higher-class, unquestionably racially white show.

Nevertheless, the very conservatism of the showgirl figure and the

Ziegfeld Girl in particular guarantees the potential of another reading altogether: the comedy and irony of camp. Camp sites are power sites, after all, spaces where dominant meanings and values are challenged and "sent up." As I pointed out in my introduction, Ziegfeld Girls are gloriously reproduced as drag queens in Howard Crabtree's 1993 *Whoop-Dee-Doo!,* and as retro nostalgia and burlesque in Madonna's *Girlie Show;* John Lahr's mother is publicized as a former Ziegfeld Girl, but so is Dorothy McHugh, star of the infamous "I've fallen and I can't get up" television ad. Nostalgia—for reckless consumption and unambiguous meanings of women—morphs quickly into camp.

The images from the 1930s and 1940s films are endlessly camp-comic in their very excesses and seriousness: Ziegfeld as the god and ringmaster of showgirls; hundreds of chorines in feathers, beads, and wigs with sequin tendrils; bejeweled women with shrubbery growing out of their headdresses. The earnestness of the Ziegfeld enterprise—its grand investment in the props, bodies, and costumes meant to awe and amaze—slips all too easily into bathos. Similarly, Verhoeven's *Showgirls,* with its ambitiously steamy sexuality, quickly became fodder for camp readings. *Showgirls'* protagonist Nomi rises from strip club lap dancer to star of a specifically Ziegfeldesque Las Vegas casino show called *Goddess.* In the film's most-quoted, not-intentionally-funny scenes, Nomi licks poles in her dance routine at the low-class Cheetah Club as a sign of primitive animal sexuality, whereas in the high-class *Goddess,* she gyrates in front of a papier-mâché volcano as a sign of imaginative, big-money sexuality. The film's serious offerings of X-rated sex, especially in conjunction with its deadpan redux of *All about Eve* backstage jealousy, were the very terms of its campy reception.

Current debates about the political value of camp, particularly its identities with queer politics and its alignment with or against feminism, offer rich rereadings of Ziegfeldian theater. From the perspective of camp, the most repressive aspects of the Ziegfeld Walk, choreography, and discipline can be turned topsy-turvy, as revelations that neither haute couture fashion nor the statuesque feminine body need necessarily be female or heterosexual. Moreover, the assumption that camp appeals primarily to gay men has come under question recently, with discussion of a "feminist camp" that can highlight "how women have negotiated their feelings of alienation from the normative gender and sex roles assigned to them by straight culture," as Pamela Robertson puts it.[6] The basics of camp—as both politics and style—also foreground and, for my purposes here, neatly summarize basic assumptions of the Ziegfeld enterprise that made it so successful and so enduring.

First, Ziegfeld's claim that he "invented" the showgirl and the subsequent cultural acknowledgments of Ziegfeld as an "originator" of female glamour set up the Ziegfeld enterprise as an "original" image. Authenticity of jewelry and fine fabric on the Ziegfeld stage supposedly signified an authenticity of body, gender, and sexuality as well, hooking this coherent identity to a classed and racialized economy. The Glorified American Girl as an original, authentic body acquired authority and privilege, helping to map out the terrain of other bodies as less visible and less important. Camp parody has political pungency because it calls the bluff on the original as less than inevitable.[7] Drag queens paying homage to Ziegfeld Girls in *Whoop-Dee-Doo!* undercut a presumed coherency of gender, sexuality, and clothing. The context of the parody is gay male culture, but the definitions of the privileged "original" are so narrow and constraining—female heterosexuality as a specific age and body that looks good in push-up bras and feathers—that a far wider cultural audience has a stake in this parody's humor.

Second, camp as a mode of rereading exposes the contradictions of bourgeois respectability, the essence of Ziegfeldness that was already on wobbly legs in the two Leonard films, *The Great Ziegfeld* biopic and *Ziegfeld Girl*. The niceness of the Ziegfeld Girl, her status as household pet, in its logical extreme suggests female sexuality at the cheerful service of male needs and desires. In Leonard's biopic, the weak link is Ziegfeld as genius producer of showgirls and Ziegfeld as dirty old man; Ziegfeld's serious lecture to little Mary Lou about how he loves all the little girls and her reappearance as mature showgirl ready to sit in his lap are perfectly awful in their cornball defensiveness. In *Ziegfeld Girl*, one of the camp exposures is the appearance of twenty sumptuous brass beds on which twenty Ziegfeld Girls do a dance routine in the final production number, hinting at the Ziegfeld Girls' actual use value, spelled out in the Lana Turner subplot.

Finally, camp readings seize on rigid and excessive definitions, especially rigid definitions of sexuality and gender, as reversible and thus ironic and potentially comic. The gender/sexuality excesses of melodrama are particularly vulnerable to camp laughter, evident in any viewing of the *Glorifying the American Girl* finale, in which Gloria miserably, bravely accepts her fate as star of the Ziegfeld stage, wearing a six-foot feather chandelier on her head and surrounded by giant jeweled butterflies, while her true love dotes on his less frightening brunette wife in the audience. The visual excesses of the Ziegfeld style similarly call attention to themselves as trying too hard, working too obviously at "real" glamour or "real" sexuality. In a Busby Berkeley number such as "In the Money" from *Gold Diggers,* women's bodies are set up as riches but also as physically impossible entities (hundreds of sparkling legs and gold-coin chests), so that female heterosexuality is overdefined into virtual meaninglessness. Likewise Dick Powell's voyeuristic daydream in *Footlight Parade*'s "By a Waterfall" multiplies one splashing woman into fountains of identical women and into explicit lesbian images, the women linked and swimming happily between each other's legs. When Powell reappears and reclaims the heterosexual meaning of the dream with an image of a cozy bird family in its nest, the result is inadvertently hilarious.

Judy Garland figures in these trying-too-hard images of Ziegfeldness in two 1940s representations that contribute to her own camp appeal. In *Ziegfeld Girl,* her costumes take on a life of their own (the palm tree hat in "Minnie" evolves into the blond, sausage-curl wig in the finale) to fill the gap between Garland and her glamorous Ziegfeld persona. Garland also appears in a comic number of *The Ziegfeld Follies* (1946), the Vincente Minnelli revue reenactment, as the Great Lady with her gay male entourage.[8] This mockery of classic female stardom exaggerates its plush accessories and self-dramatized posing, both of which also characterized the classic Ziegfeld Girl. The later film allows Garland to clown around with the ideal, camping up the image that the Leonard film asks us to take seriously, although this seriousness itself offers camp readings and distance.

Garland's famous uneasiness with stardom and glamour, the doubleness of her performances that has made her particularly beloved to gay male culture, has special resonance in the meanings of the Ziegfeld enterprise. The Ziegfeld Girl's perfect composure aimed to make feminine disciplines look easy. In *Ziegfeld Girl*'s "You Stepped Out of a Dream Number," the women glide down staircases with apparent effortlessness, even though a previous scene showed them rehearsing the Walk while straining to balance hefty telephone books on their heads.

In contrast to dreamy Ziegfeld Girl gliding, Garland's performances make heterosexuality look difficult — explaining why straight women, as well as gay men, would find Garland appealing as camp.[9] When Garland enacts the Ziegfeld Girl, the seams show. The material tugs at tight spots. Perhaps she is the essence of Ziegfeldness after all. The final image of the Leonard film, with the blond-wigged Garland as the top-of-the-wedding-cake Ziegfeld Girl, is ludicrous and cruel but also beloved in its failure to fill an impossible, sadly narrow ideal. The image painfully wedges open the chasm between ordinary life and the realm of Ziegfeldian showcasing, like John Lahr's stories about his mother or my own observations of the stately Lina Basquette.

NOTEſ

Introduction: Glory, Legend, ant the Ziegfeld Guarantee

1. Douglas Martin, "The Choreography of Desire: Ex-Follies Girl Recalls Glory Days," *New York Times*, 18 Oct. 1996, sec. A; "1000 Makers of Music," *London Sunday Times*, Special Sections, Oct.–Nov. 1997.

2. Percy Hammond, "Let Us All Stand while the Coryphees Sing 'Oh, Say,'" *Chicago Tribune*, 5 Dec. 1915.

3. "Ziegfeld Trade-Mark Asset to Chorus Girl: Means Beauty, Youth, Animation, Stage Sparkle, and Knack of Weaving Clothes Chic-ly," *New York Mail*, 17 July 1915.

4. Alexander Woollcott, "The Invisible Fish" (1929), reprint, *The Portable Woollcott*, ed. Joseph Hennessey (New York: Viking, 1946), 445.

5. In her treatment of Marilyn Monroe, S. Paige Baty gives a useful definition of "icons" as "circulated figures or characters that become the very surface on which other meanings are communicated. . . . [T]hey are the sites for repeated stagings of narratives, the sites on which the past, present, and future may be written." See *American Monroe: The Making of a Body Politic* (Berkeley and Los Angeles: University of California Press, 1995), 60.

6. See Arthur Frank Wertheim, ed., *Will Rogers at the Ziegfeld Follies*, (Norman: University of Oklahoma Press, 1992), 15.

7. "Funny Clowning in the Ziegfeld Follies of 1912," *New York Globe*, 22 Oct. 1912.

8. Edmund Wilson, "The Follies as an Institution" (1923), reprint, *The Portable Edmund Wilson*, ed. Lewis M. Dabney (New York: Viking, 1983), 183–84.

9. As Joan Scott has put it, the retellings of events are less important than understanding "how the subjective and collective meanings of women and men as categories of identity have been constructed." See *Gender and the Politics of History* (New York: Columbia University Press, 1988), 6. Scott points out the value of literary poststructuralism as historical methodology because it puts emphasis on "the ways arguments are structured and presented as well as to what is literally said" (7).

10. Robert C. Toll, *On with the Show: The First Century of Show Business in America* (New York: Oxford University Press, 1976), 296. See also Toll's contextualization of Ziegfeld within American show business, 295–326.

11. Ibid., 317.

12. See Peter Bailey, "Parasexuality and Glamour: The Victorian Barmaid as Cultural Prototype," *Gender and History* 2, 2 (1990): 148–72. I am indebted to Bailey for this description of "glamour" as a "modern visual property" dependent on the distance between the desired object and the smitten spectator

(152). Bailey points out that the word was introduced by Sir Walter Scott as a poetic way to describe beauty that was magical or based on illusion. The word itself comes from "grammar," meaning occult learning or rules.

13. See John Hirsch, "The American Revue Costume," in *Musical Theatre in America,* ed. Glenn Loney (Westport, Conn: Greenwood, 1984), 155.

14. Nathan Teitel, "The Man Who Invented Women," *Saturday Review,* 4 Nov. 1972, 84–86; Ignatz Jacobson, "My Wife Is a Showgirl," *Louisville Herald,* 21 Nov. 1915.

15. The Brazilian fish anecdote appears in several biographies of Ziegfeld, but without documentation, and may itself illustrate the hype of Ziegfeldian theater lore.

16. For an account of Ziegfeld's publicity as transparent, see Rennold Wolf, "The P. T. Barnum of the Theatre," *Green Book,* June 1914, 933–46.

17. Marjorie Farnsworth, *The Ziegfeld Follies: A History in Text and Pictures* (New York: Putnam's, 1956), 11.

18. Eddie Cantor and David Freedman, *Ziegfeld, the Great Glorifier* (New York: Alfred H. King, 1934), 21.

19. For details of the new theater district and its clientele, see Lewis A. Erenberg, *Steppin' Out: New York Nightlife and the Transformation of American Culture, 1890–1930* (1981; reprint, Chicago: University of Chicago Press, 1984), esp. 33–59. Gerald Mast describes the early development of the American musical-comedy tradition in *Can't Help Singin': The American Musical on Stage and Screen* (Woodstock, N.Y.: Overlook, 1987), 7–24. For a description of the American theatrical-spectacle tradition and its refinement in the revues of Ziegfeld and his colleagues, see Martin Rubin, *Showstoppers: Busby Berkeley and the Tradition of Spectacle* (New York: Columbia University Press, 1993), 14–26.

20. Liane Carrera, *Anna Held and Flo Ziegfeld* (1954), trans. Guy Daniels (Hicksville, N.Y.: Exposition, 1979), 85.

21. Liane Carrera, untitled manuscript, Anna Held Museum Papers, Billy Rose Theatre Collection, New York Public Library for the Performing Arts. The Billy Rose Theatre Collection is hereafter abbreviated as BRTC.

22. Ibid.

23. *Follies* review, *New York World,* 14 July 1907, and " 'Follies of 1909' Gets Aerial Start," *New York World,* 15 June 1909.

24. "Follies of 1909," *New York Star,* clipping, BRTC; " 'Follies' Begin Summer Capers," *New York Times,* 2 June 1914.

25. Gerald Bordman, *American Musical Revue: From the Passing Show to Sugar Babies* (New York: Oxford University Press, 1985), 36.

26. The story about Ziegfeld's time schedule for a comic sketch can be found in Randolph Carter, *Ziegfeld: The Time of His Life* (1974; reprint, London: Bernard, 1988), 77, and in Toll, *On with the Show,* 315.

27. "Lines on the Summer Revue Folk," *New York Times,* 16 Aug. 1931; J. P. McEvoy, "He Knew What They Wanted," *Saturday Evening Post,* 10 Sept. 1932, 10.

28. Hugh Fordin, *Getting to Know Him: A Biography of Oscar Hammerstein II* (New York: Random House, 1977), 85, and Gilbert Seldes, "The Great Glorifier" (1931), reprint, *New Yorker*, 31 May 1993, 60.

29. Ed Sullivan, "Broadway," *Pittsburgh Press*, 11 Apr. 1936.

30. "Men behind the Plays," *New York Times*, 11 Feb. 1923; George J. Nathan, "Ziegfeld" (1923), reprint, *The Magic Mirror* (New York: Alfred A. Knopf, 1960), 90, 89; McEvoy, "He Knew What They Wanted."

31. George Brenton Beak, "Follies Glorify Girlish Beauty," *Boston Post*, 3 Aug. 1927; "Pittsburgh Grows Follies Conscious," *Post-Gazette*, 15 June 1931; Seldes, "The Great Glorifier," 60.

32. J. Brooks Atkinson, "The Play: The Follies Comes of Age," *New York Times*, 17 Aug. 1927.

33. Ted LeBerthon, "Ziegfeld Follies," *Los Angeles Record*, 28 Apr. 1930. See also George Jean Nathan, "Ziegfeld and His Follies Win International Reputation," *Judge*, 25 Aug. 1923.

34. Cantor and Freedman, *Ziegfeld, the Great Glorifier*, 9.

35. See Adele Rogers St. John, "The Girls Who Glorified Ziegfeld," *American Weekly*, 7 July 1946; "Ziegfeld's Girls Hold a Reunion," *Life*, 13 Dec. 1948; and Bernard Sobel, "This Was Ziegfeld," *American Mercury*, Jan. 1945, 96–102.

36. Farnsworth, *The Ziegfeld Follies*, 84.

37. This "call" suggests Louis Althusser's well-known trope for the efficacy and invisibility of ideology, the power of ideology to seem obvious and commonsensical. When addressed by cultural texts as "You," we respond as the one being "hailed," so that what is constructed looks natural or what has been formulated seems inevitable. Althusser describes ideology not as manipulative rigging behind the scenes but as embedded in "obviousnesses which we cannot fail to recognize," so that our response is " 'That's obvious! That's right! That's true!' " See "Ideology and Ideological State Apparatuses," in *Lenin and Philosophy, and Other Essays*, trans. Ben Brewster (New York: Monthly Review, 1971), 172.

38. Robert Baral, "Ziegfeld and His Follies," *Variety*, 9 Jan. 1957, 295+.

39. For the homage to Ziegfeld and the Beauty Trust, see Robert Baral, *Revue: A Nostalgic Reprise of the Great Broadway Period* (New York: Fleet, 1962), 33–34. For the summary referencing the Irving Berlin tune and the "bring on the girls" illustration, see 263–64.

40. Charles Higham, *Ziegfeld* (Chicago: Regnery, 1972), 233.

41. Carter, *Ziegfeld: The Time of His Life*, 81.

42. Richard Ziegfeld and Paulette Ziegfeld, *The Ziegfeld Touch: The Life and Times of Florenz Ziegfeld, Jr.* (New York: Abrams, 1993), 178–79.

43. Michael Lasser, "The Glorifier: Florenz Ziegfeld and the Creation of the American Showgirl," *American Scholar* 63 (1994): 441, 448. Other Ziegfeld scholarly studies have provided detailed documentation of Ziegfeld's enterprise in similarly admiring terms. For full-length histories of the *Follies*, see Geraldine A. Maschio, "The Ziegfeld Follies: Form, Content, and the Signifi-

cance of an American Revue" (Ph.D. diss., University of Wisconsin-Madison, 1981), and Rosaline B. Stone, "The Ziegfeld Follies: A Study of Theatrical Opulence from 1907 to 1931" (Ph.D. diss., University of Denver, 1985).

44. "Ziegfeld: Glorifying the British Musical?" *Theater Week*, 4–10 July 1988, 41.

45. Laura Mulvey, "Visual Pleasure and Narrative Cinema," *Screen* 16 (1975): 13–14. Since its publication, this argument has been very much refined and qualified by Mulvey herself and many others. It remains a powerful touchstone not only for feminist film theory but also generally for its ability to explain the dynamics of female spectacle in a number of visual texts.

46. Rick Altman, *The American Film Musical* (Bloomington: Indiana University Press, 1987), 243. See also Mast's descriptions of Ziegfeld's influence on movie musicals in *Can't Help Singin'*, 116–17, 121.

47. Toll postulates that show business women of this era, from serious actress to showgirls, may themselves have continued the threat of "highly visible, 'racy,' liberated women." See *On with the Show*, 245.

48. See Richard Dyer, *Heavenly Bodies: Film Stars and Society* (New York: St. Martin's, 1986), 17.

49. William R. Leach, *Land of Desire: Merchants, Power, and the Rise of a New American Culture* (New York: Pantheon, 1993), 9, and Robert C. Allen, *Horrible Prettiness: Burlesque and American Culture* (Chapel Hill: University of North Carolina Press, 1991), 245. For a description of the new consumer and her desires, see Rachel Bowlby, *Just Looking: Consumer Culture in Dreiser, Gissing, and Zola* (New York: Methuen, 1985), 1–17.

50. See Theodore E. Allen, *The Invention of the White Race* (London: Verso, 1994). For a study of whiteness and white women in British culture, see Vron Ware, *Beyond the Pale: White Women, Racism, and History* (London: Verso, 1992). See also Ruth Frankenberg's sociological study of racial and sexual relations, *White Women, Race Matters: The Social Construction of Whiteness* (Minneapolis: University of Minnesota Press, 1993).

51. Laura Doyle, *Bordering on the Body: The Racial Matrix of Modern Fiction and Culture* (New York: Oxford University Press, 1994), 26. Doyle emphasizes that "hierarchies of race and gender require one another as co-originating and co-dependent forms of oppression rather than merely parallel, compounded, or intersecting forms" (21).

52. Richard Dyer, *White* (London: Routledge, 1997), 25, 47.

53. See Martha Banta, *Imaging American Women: Idea and Ideals in Cultural History* (New York: Columbia University Press, 1987), and Lois W. Banner, *American Beauty* (New York: Knopf, 1983).

54. See Robert C. Allen, *Horrible Prettiness*, in particular chap. 2, "The Intelligibility of Burlesque," 25–42. See also Allen on the Ziegfeld Girl, 245–46, 272, 282.

55. Erenberg, *Steppin' Out*, bibliographical essay.

56. Charles Higham, *Ziegfeld*, 29; Toll, *On with the Show*, 317. Teresa de Lauretis

revises Foucault's concept of a "technology of sex," the institutionalized discourses shaping sexual behaviors, by specifying how such technologies affect women and men differently. See de Lauretis, "The Technology of Gender," in *Technologies of Gender: Essays on Theory, Film, and Fiction* (Bloomington: Indiana University Press, 1987), 1–30.

57. Michel Foucault, *The History of Sexuality: An Introduction*, vol. 1 of *The History of Sexuality*, trans. Robert Hurley (1978; reprint, New York: Vintage, 1990), 147, 97.

58. Elizabeth Grosz, *Volatile Bodies: Toward a Corporeal Feminism* (Bloomington: Indiana University Press, 1994), 23.

1. Celebrity and Glamour: Anna Held

1. Lois W. Banner makes this point about the later popular image of the beauty in the bubble bath. See *American Beauty*, 186. See also Banner's account of the proliferation of female images of sensuality and sexuality at the turn of the century, 184–87.

2. *New York World*, 9 May 1897, Robinson Locke Collection Scrapbook 264, BRTC.

3. Richard deCordova, *Picture Personalities: The Emergence of the Star System in America* (Urbana: University of Illinois Press, 1990), 141. For another excellent example of stardom scholarship that reads body and persona as cultural text, see Ramona Curry, *Too Much of a Good Thing: Mae West as Cultural Icon* (Minneapolis: University of Minnesota Press, 1996).

4. Cantor and Freedman, *Ziegfeld, the Great Glorifier*, 33.

5. "Anna Held Frowns on Hypocrisy," *Los Angeles Examiner*, 3 Jan. 1912. See also the extensive clippings from nationwide newspapers in the Robinson Locke Collection Scrapbooks 264 and 266, BRTC.

6. For the *New York Times* coverage of Held's personal life, see, for example, "Mlle. Anna Held Arrives," 16 Sept. 1896; "Anna Held to be Married," 7 Jan. 1897; "Denies the Engagement: Manager Ziegfeld Says That He Is Not to Marry Anna Held," 8 Jan. 1897; "Anna Held Sues for Divorce," 14 Apr. 1912.

7. See Channing Pollock, *Harvest of My Years: An Autobiography* (Indianapolis: Bobbs-Merrill, 1943), 123–24. According to Bernard Sobel, another of Ziegfeld's publicists, the barrage of fake stories from Ziegfeld's publicity office often took on a life of their own, so that Ziegfeld himself was at times mistaken about the truth of *Follies* "news" stories. "He was taken in, time after time, by the very publicity he authorized," Sobel points out (Sobel, "This Was Ziegfeld," 99). For the influence of P. T. Barnum in the celebrity business, especially in the "creation" of news, see Leo Braudy, *The Frenzy of Renown: Fame and Its History* (New York: Oxford University Press, 1986), 498–506, and Joshua Gamson, *Claims to Fame: Celebrity in Contemporary America* (Berkeley: University of California Press, 1994), 22–23.

8. Gamson, *Claims to Fame*, 141.

9. Woollcott, "The Invisible Fish," 451.

10. See Carrera, *Anna Held and Flo Ziegfeld*, 71–72, 85. The Bennett story is reported by Woollcott, ibid., 450–51.

11. See "Miss Anna Held Hurt," *New York Times*, 19 Oct. 1896, and " 'Heroines' and Press Agents," *New York Times*, 20 Oct. 1896; James S. Metcalfe, "The Stage and the Beauty Problem," *Cosmopolitan*, Nov. 1896; and *Cincinnati Commercial*, 3 July 1910.

12. Lisa Duggan cites the notoriety of French fiction for Americans in the 1890s in "The Trials of Alice Mitchell: Sensationalism, Sexology, and the Lesbian Subject in Turn-of-the-Century America," *Signs* 18, 4 (1993): 791–814.

13. Carrera, *Anna Held and Flo Ziegfeld*, 115.

14. As Maureen Turim has pointed out, for Americans of that era, "the attraction of continental sophistication for an upwardly mobile bourgeoisie was enormous." See "Seduction and Elegance: The New Woman of Fashion in Silent Cinema," in *On Fashion*, ed. Shari Benstock and Suzanne Ferriss (New Brunswick, N.J.: Rutgers University Press, 1994), 147.

15. "Anna Held Illustrates How to Lace Tight," "My Philosophy of Dress," "The Parisian Woman," "May Graduate to Jeweled Corset Hooks Themselves," "My Own Beauty Secrets," and many other articles featuring Held's advice on corsetry fashion can be found in the Robinson Locke Collection Scrapbooks 264 and 266, BRTC.

16. Anna Held, supposedly quoted in an interview, "May Graduate to Jeweled Corset Hooks Themselves," *Cleveland News*, 26 Dec. 1907.

17. See Patricia Ziegfeld, *The Ziegfelds' Girl: Confessions of an Abnormally Happy Childhood* (Boston: Little, Brown, 1964), 44. Marjorie Farnsworth also reports this story in *The Ziegfeld Follies*, 30. Billie Burke, in contrast, reports in her autobiography that Anna Held died as a result of excessive dieting "in an effort to recapture her great beauty." See *With a Feather on My Nose* (New York: Appleton-Century-Crofts, 1949), 144.

18. Jacques-Charles, foreword to Carrera, *Anna Held and Flo Ziegfeld*, 7.

19. Casey Finch, " 'Hooked and Buttoned Together': Victorian Underwear and Representations of the Female Body," *Victorian Studies* 34, 3 (1991): 337–63. See Finch's discussion of the shift from belly to hourglass, 340–43. See also David Kunzle, "Dress Reform as Antifeminism: A Response to Helene E. Robert's 'The Exquisite Slave: The Role of Clothing in the Making of the Victorian Woman,' " *Signs* 2, 3 (1977): 570–79. The meanings of corsetry have been hotly debated in feminist and cultural studies. For an excellent summary of these debates, see Jennifer Craik, *The Face of Fashion: Cultural Studies in Fashion* (London: Routledge, 1994), 119–26; quotation is from page 125.

20. *New York World*, 27 Dec. 1906, and Carrera, *Anna Held and Flo Ziegfeld*, 165.

21. Carrera, *Anna Held and Flo Ziegfeld*, 101.

22. John D'Emilio and Estelle B. Freedman, *Intimate Matters: A History of Sexuality in America* (New York: Harper and Row, 1988), 181. For the statistics on venereal disease, see 183.

23. Eugene Lemoyne Connelly, "Anna Held Would Make Marriage Compulsory," *Pittsburgh Leader,* Apr. 1914.

24. Untitled newspaper clipping, Robinson Locke Collection Scrapbook 266, BRTC. In the same scrapbook, see "All the Votes for Men, All the Love for Women: Anne Held's Creed," *Chicago Examiner,* 2 Jan. 1910.

25. Carrera, *Anna Held and Flo Ziegfeld,* 114.

26. For an excellent study of this female gaze produced by novelties in nineteenth-century visual experience, see Anne Friedberg, *Window Shopping: Cinema and the Postmodern* (Berkeley: University of California Press, 1993), 32–37, 47–94.

27. "And Now They All Want Oriental Eyes," *New York World,* 20 Jan. 1907.

28. Charles Higham, *Ziegfeld,* 25–26.

29. See Lulla Adler Rosenfeld, *The Yiddish Theatre and Jacob P. Adler,* 2d ed. (New York: Shapolsky, 1988), 185–86.

30. Held's "Polish Jewish parentage" is correctly identified by the *New York Times* article announcing her engagement, "Anna Held to be Married," 7 Jan. 1897, but most other *Times* articles refer to her as "the French actress." See also "Anna Held's Real Nativity," March 1899, unmarked clipping, Robinson Locke Collection Scrapbook 266, BRTC, a newspaper article entertaining rumors "that Anna Held is not a French woman, but a Hungarian Jewess."

31. "Anna Held Still American," *New York Times,* 7 Nov. 1915.

32. See Peter Stallybrass and Allon White, *The Politics and Poetics of Transgression* (Ithaca, N.Y.: Cornell University Press, 1986), esp. on hybridization and the grotesque, 112–18 and 193–202, respectively.

33. Pamela Brown, "Coon Shouting and the Americanization of the Jewish Ziegfeld Girl," unpublished seminar paper, New York University, 1994. I am enormously indebted to Pamela Brown for her extensive work on Anna Held's Jewish identity and Held's work within the coon-shouting tradition. Brown postulates that coon shouting may have been an assimilation device for Jews at the turn of the century. See also Peter Stanfield's description of coon songs in " 'An Octoroon in the Kindling': American Vernacular and Blackface Minstrelsy in 1930s Hollywood," *Journal of American Studies* 31 (1997): 417–19.

34. Carrera, *Anna Held and Flo Ziegfeld,* 91.

35. Ibid.

36. See Eric Lott, *Love and Theft: Blackface Minstrelsy and the American Working Class* (New York: Oxford University Press, 1993), especially 147–50.

37. *Newark Star,* 15 July 1918. For other examples of Burke's star persona as domestic sweetheart, see Billie Burke, "On Acting and Babies," *American Magazine,* Aug. 1918, 58–59; Billie Burke, "Billie Burke Remembers," *Delineator,* June 1924, 12+; "Billie Burke, Married and at Home," *Green Book,* Nov. 1914, 843–54; Alan Dale, "Billie Burke, Comedienne," *Cosmopolitan,* May 1914, 842–44.

38. Carrera, *Anna Held and Flo Ziegfeld,* 175.

39. The museum guide, the manuscripts, and Ginger Rogers's reply to Carrera's letter are in the Anna Held Museum Papers, BRTC. Four typewritten manuscripts and a play synopsis seem to be variations of the published book. The

author of each is designated Liane Carrera or "Anna Held Jr." Richard and Paulette Ziegfeld point out a number of additional problems in accepting Held's memoirs as anything but Carrera's. See *The Ziegfeld Touch*, 39, 45.

40. Carrera, *Anna Held and Flo Ziegfeld*, 121.
41. "Anna Held Not Rehearsed," *New York Times*, 6 Sept. 1913.
42. "Anna Held's Debut in a Screen Play," *New York Times*, 7 Feb. 1916; "Anna Held Hears Last Curtain Rung," *New York Times*, 27 May 1918. Pamela Brown cites the Joan of Arc speech as part of Held's identity contentions in "Coon Shouting and the Americanization of the Jewish Ziegfeld Girl."

2. Chorus Girls, New Women, True Bodies

1. "A Chorus Girl Factory," *New York American*, 20 June 1909.
2. Lois W. Banner uses these estimates in *American Beauty*, 183.
3. Kathy Peiss, *Cheap Amusements: Working Women and Leisure in Turn-of-the-Century New York* (Philadelphia: Temple University Press, 1986), 7. See also Banner's description of this social and recreational shift in *American Beauty*, 175–201.
4. See Erenberg, *Steppin' Out*, chap. 3, "Women Out of Control: Critics of the New Amusements," 60–110. See also chap. 7, "Broadway Babies: Glorifying the American Girl, 1915–1922," 206–30, for an excellent description of the chorus girl in cabaret culture and Ziegfeld's contributions to the development of cabaret.
5. For example, historian Christina Simmons argues that the stereotype of the asexual Victorian woman was part of a larger strategy to contain and control female sexuality just at the moment when birth control was becoming available and women were being encouraged to express their sexuality in marriage. Describing the emergence of the flapper as social ideal in the 1920s, Simmons emphasizes that this youthful, sexualized figure was often contrasted to the repressed Victorian matron, in 1920s media, for curious reasons. The flapper, after all, was hardly a sexually threatening presence, suggesting instead that "a youthful and malleable adolescent was more attractive than a sexually experienced adult woman." See "Modern Sexuality and the Myth of Victorian Repression," in *Passion and Power: Sexuality in History*, ed. Kathy Peiss and Christina Simmons (Philadelphia: Temple University Press, 1989), 169.
6. Erenberg, *Steppin' Out*, 215, 206.
7. P. G. Wodehouse and Guy Bolton, *Bring On the Girls! The Improbable Story of Our Life in Musical Comedy* (New York: Simon and Schuster, 1953), 152.
8. Robert C. Allen, *Horrible Prettiness*, 96. Benjamin McArthur, *Actors and American Culture, 1880–1920* (Philadelphia: Temple University Press, 1984), 15–16.
9. See, for example, "The Experiences of a Chorus Girl," *Independent*, 12 July 1906, 80–85; Alice Francis, "The Woes of a Chorus Girl," *Green Book*, May 1909, 968–71; Will Livingston Agnew, "Puck's Understudy: A Chorus Girl's

Big Opportunity," *Green Book*, Apr. 1910, 820–22; Newton A. Fuessle, "The Clergyman and the Chorus Girl," *Green Book*, Oct. 1911, 810–16; Margaret McIvor-Tyndall, "The Truth about the Chorus Girl," *Dance Lovers Magazine*, Apr. 1924, 14.

10. Alan Dale, "Among Other Things," *Variety*, 6 Oct. 1916, 2.

11. *American*, 13 June 1910 and 20 June 1921, and the *New York World*, 27 Dec. 1906.

12. See McCardell's columns in the *New York World*, 27 Dec. 1906, 13 Jan. 1907, 18 Aug. 1907, and 29 May 1910.

13. Madge Merton, *Confessions of a Chorus Girl* (New York: Grafton, 1903), 42, 52–53.

14. Roy L. McCardell, *Conversations of a Chorus Girl* (New York: Street and Smith, 1903), 17–18, 121–22.

15. Bailey, "Parasexuality and Glamour," 166, 163.

16. Laurence Senelick, "Private Parts in Public Places," in *Inventing Times Square: Commerce and Culture at the Crossroads of the World*, ed. William R. Taylor (New York: Russell Sage, 1991), 331.

17. For more on this new female visibility and its ambivalences, see Anne Friedberg, *Window Shopping*, 32–37. See also Constance Balides, "Scenarios of Exposure in the Practice of Everyday Life: Women in the Cinema of Attractions," *Screen* 34, 1 (1993): 19–37, on the social surveillance that read sexuality in "the everyday" because of this new visibility.

18. For a description of this "sporting male" culture, see Timothy J. Gilfoyle, "Policing of Sexuality," in *Inventing Times Square*, ed. Taylor, 297–314.

19. See Senelick, "Private Parts in Public Places," 331.

20. These quotations from Avery Hopwood's *Gold Diggers* appear respectively in Arthur Hove, "Introduction: In Search of Happiness," in *Gold Diggers of 1933*, ed. Arthur Hove (Madison: University of Wisconsin Press, 1980), 10, and in Jack F. Sharrar, *Avery Hopwood: His Life and Plays* (Jefferson, N. C.: McFarland, 1989), 115.

21. See Mary P. Ryan, *Womanhood in America: From Colonial Times to the Present* (New York: Franklin Watts, 1983), 200–210.

22. See Susan Porter Benson, *Counter Cultures: Saleswomen, Managers, and Customers in American Department Stores, 1890–1940* (Urbana: University of Illinois Press, 1986). For a study of pink-collar work, see Sharon Hartman Strom, *Beyond the Typewriter: Gender, Class, and the Origins of Modern American Office Work* (Urbana: University of Illinois Press, 1992). See also Susan A. Glenn's study of working-class women, *Daughters of the Shtetl: Life and Labor in the Immigrant Generation* (Ithaca, N.Y.: Cornell University Press, 1990).

23. James S. Metcalfe, "The Why of the Chorus Girl," *Theatre Magazine*, Apr. 1921, 248.

24. Concerning this supposed modern freedom, Martin Pumphrey comments that the modern housewife and the 1920s flapper were, ironically, produced in the same continuum, targeted by advertising that convinced them their

individuality could be achieved only through the purchase of particular com-modities. See "The Flapper, the Housewife, and the Making of Modernity," *Cultural Studies* 1 (1987): 179–94.

25. Suzannah Lessard, "Stanford White's Ruins," *New Yorker,* 8 July 1996, 49–65. See also Martha Banta's comments on Nesbit in *Imaging American Women,* 664–66, and Michael MacDonald Mooney, *Evelyn Nesbit and Stanford White: Love and Death in the Gilded Age* (New York: William Morrow, 1976).

26. See Banner's discussion of the Gibson Girl in *American Beauty,* 154–74. The Gibson Girl, she points out, was "a fantasy figure in whom the problems of poverty, immigration, and labor strife were denied" (169). Banta's *Imaging American Women* details the vast array of contradictory popular images of the New Woman, but see in particular the illustrations in chap. 1, "American Girls and the New Woman," 45–91.

27. *The American Girl As Seen and Portrayed by Howard Chandler Christy* (New York: Moffat, Yard, and Company, 1906), 12, 20.

28. *New York World,* 16 Aug. 1907.

29. "The Gibson Bathing Girl," music by Alfred Solman, lyrics by Paul West (Joseph W. Stern and Company, 1907).

30. "Observe the Gibson Curve," *New York World,* 4 Aug. 1907.

31. This description of the 1909 *Follies* comes from Joseph Kaye, "Master of the Follies," *Dance Magazine,* Dec. 1929, 34.

32. Louis Sherwin, "Musical Comedy and the Drier Drama," *Vanity Fair,* Feb. 1917, 59+.

33. For the turn-of-the-century New Woman as "portrait of evil," see Bram Dijk-stra, *Idols of Perversity: Fantasies of Feminine Evil in Fin-de-Siècle Culture* (New York: Oxford University Press, 1986).

34. "That Ragtime Suffragette," Harry Williams and Nat. D. Ayer (New York: Harry Williams Music Company, 1913).

35. "The Vampire," by Earl Jones, Gene Buck, and Bert A. Williams (New York: Jerome H. Remick and Company, 1913).

36. Florenz Ziegfeld Jr., "Picking Out Pretty Girls for the Stage," *American Maga-zine,* Dec. 1919, 34+.

37. Cantor and Freedman, *Ziegfeld, the Great Glorifier,* 45–46.

38. Arthur Lubow, *The Reporter Who Would Be King: A Biography of Richard Hard-ing Davis* (New York: Scribner's, 1992), 126.

39. Ibid., 229.

40. Ibid., 267.

41. Ibid., 330.

42. Ibid., 330. Clippings file for Bessie McCoy, no source or date, BRTC.

43. Banta, *Imaging American Women,* 273, 275.

44. For cross-dressing as symptom of category crisis, see Marjorie Garber, *Vested Interests: Cross-Dressing and Cultural Anxiety* (1992; reprint, New York: Harper-Perennial, 1993).

45. Historians and scholars of sexuality have long debated the actual effects of

the medical namings and categorizations of homosexuality/heterosexuality late in the nineteenth century. For an extended discussion of the development of these terms, see Jonathan Ned Katz, *The Invention of Heterosexuality* (New York: Dutton, 1995), 19–32.

46. The question of how to name these relationships is a complex one and be-yond the scope of this study. See Lillian Faderman, *Surpassing the Love of Men: Romantic Friendship and Love between Women from the Renaissance to the Present* (New York: Quill, 1981), 311–13, 328–31, 411–15.

47. According to George Chauncey, "The medical analysis of the different char-acter of 'inverts,' 'perverts,' and 'normal people' reflected a set of classificatory distinctions already widely recognized in the broader culture." See *Gay New York: Gender, Urban Culture, and the Making of the Gay Male World, 1890–1940* (New York: Basic, 1994), 125. For Chauncey's discussion of the impact of the "fairy" on the forging of middle-class masculinity, see 111–16.

48. As Terry Castle has put it, "When it comes to lesbians . . . many people have trouble seeing what's in front of them." See *The Apparitional Lesbian: Female Homosexuality and Modern Culture* (New York: Columbia University Press, 1993), 2. Castle argues that the lesbian was not an invention of turn-of-the-century sexologists but has existed as a "ghosted" figure in history, art, and literature for centuries.

49. Richard von Krafft-Ebing, *Psychopathia Sexualis* (1906; reprint, New York: Physicians and Surgeons Book Company, 1926), 398. See his chapter "Con-genital Sexual Inversion in Woman," 395–443. Havelock Ellis, *Studies in the Psychology of Sex: Sexual Inversion* (1901; reprint, Philadelphia: F. A. Davis, 1929), 222–23.

50. Carroll Smith-Rosenberg makes this point in *Disorderly Conduct: Visions of Gender in Victorian America* (New York: Knopf, 1985), 275.

51. Faderman, *Surpassing the Love of Men*, 297–99.

52. Smith-Rosenberg reminds us that this medical vocabulary was an index of considerable social and sexual uncertainty. Terms such as "the intermedi-ate sex" and "sexual inversion" "are spatial and hierarchical images, con-cerned with issues of order, structure, and difference," she writes. They imply other disturbing metaphors such as "The-Woman-on-Top" and "The-World-Upside-Down"—that is, the sexual images are images of gender roles in tran-sition. See *Disorderly Conduct*, 286.

53. "Though lesbianism as a category was partly created by sexologists, some women eagerly claimed it as their own," historians Rayna Rapp and Ellen Ross report, "for it provided a sphere in which women could both assert their social independence from men and develop a woman-centered eroticism." See Rapp and Ross, "The Twenties' Backlash: Compulsory Heterosexuality, the Consumer Family, and the Waning of Feminism," in *Class, Race, and Sex: The Dynamics of Control*, ed. Amy Swerdlow and Hanna Lessinger (Boston: G. K. Hall, 1983), 101.

54. Barry Paris, *Louise Brooks* (New York: Knopf, 1989), 419, 239. For a discussion of

strategies available to lesbians in less avant-garde circles during this time, see Lisa Duggan, "The Social Enforcement of Heterosexuality and Lesbian Resistance in the 1920s," in *Class, Race, and Sex*, ed. Swerdlow and Lessinger, 75–92.

55. Andrea Weiss, *Vampires and Violets: Lesbians in Film* (New York: Penguin, 1992), 24.

56. Kaier Curtin makes this point in *"We Can Always Call Them Bulgarians": The Emergence of Lesbians and Gay Men on the American Stage* (Boston: Alyson, 1987), 56–57.

57. See, for example, Christina Simmons, "Companionate Marriage and the Lesbian Threat," *Frontiers* 4, 3 (1979): 54–59. See also Duggan, "Social Enforcement of Heterosexuality," 75–92.

3. Costume and Choreography: Fashioning a Body

1. "The Hard Work That Goes to Make Up a Frothy Show," *Cleveland Plain Dealer*, 7 Nov. 1915.

2. J. Brooks Atkinson, "The Follies Finally Attains Its Majority," *New York Times*, 18 Sept. 1927.

3. J. Brooks Atkinson, "A New Theatrical Season Slowly Gathers Momentum," *New York Times*, 28 Aug. 1927.

4. Richard Ohmann describes this new consumerist literacy in "History and Literary History: The Case of Mass Culture," in *Modernity and Mass Culture*, ed. James Naremore and Patrick Brantlinger (Bloomington: Indiana University Press, 1991), 24–41.

5. "Ziegfeld Trade-Mark Asset to Chorus Girl," *New York Mail*, 17 July 1915.

6. "Mr. Ziegfeld and His Follies," *New York Times*, 18 June 1916.

7. "Chorus Conditions: Famous Ziegfeld Beauties Deny Allegations Affecting Their Profession," *New York Mail*, 18 Aug 1919. On the function of fashion as differentiation, see Bernard Barber and Lyle S. Lobel, " 'Fashion' in Women's Clothes and the American Social System," *Social Forces* 31, 2 (1952): 124–31.

8. John Robert Powers, *The Powers Girls: The Story of Models and Modeling and the Natural Steps by Which Attractive Girls Are Created* (New York: E. P. Dutton, 1941), 25.

9. In *The American Film Musical*, Rick Altman points out the relative novelty of "entertainment" as a passive activity in the early years of the twentieth century: "More and more, it was necessary to be entertained in order to have a good time. The concentration of pleasure in the senses of sight and hearing is nowhere more obvious than in the development of the fashionable nightclub as a place where entertainment is served up with the same style and on the same drop-in basis as the food" (204).

10. See Baral, *Revue*, 21–22.

11. J. Brooks Atkinson, "The Play," *New York Times*, 2 July 1931.

12. Liane Carrera, "Anna Held's Great Ziegfeld Folly," manuscript, Anna Held Museum Papers, BRTC.

13. The attribution to Lederer is given, for example, in "Is a 'Chorus Girl' or a 'Show Girl' an Actress?" *New York World*, 2 July 1905.

14. "New York Has Its Moulin Rouge," *New York Times*, 12 Apr. 1912.

15. Barbara Naomi Cohen-Stratyner describes this choreography in "Welcome to 'Laceland': An Analysis of a Chorus Number from the Ziegfeld Follies of 1922, as Staged by Ned Wayburn," in *Musical Theatre in America*, ed. Glenn Loney (Westport, Conn.: Greenwood, 1984), 315-22. Cohen's dissertation, "The Dance Direction of Ned Wayburn: Selected Topics in Musical Staging, 1901-1923" (Ph.D. diss., New York University, 1980), is the source of my account of Wayburn's dance innovations in the *Follies*.

16. Meredith Etherington-Smith and Jeremy Pilcher, *The "It" Girls: Lucy, Lady Duff Gordon, the Couturière "Lucile," and Elinor Glyn, Romantic Novelist* (San Diego: Harcourt Brace, 1986), 178.

17. See "The Real Reasons Agile Feet Outdistance Stately Beauty," *American*, 11 June 1916. The quotation about showgirls who can sing, dance, and talk is in "My Wife Is a Showgirl," *Louisville Herald*, 21 Nov. 1915. The interview about Ziegfeld favoring the showgirls over chorus girls backstage is quoted in Ziegfeld and Ziegfeld, *The Ziegfeld Touch*, 254-56.

18. Florenz Ziegfeld Jr., "Beauty, the Fashions, and the Follies," *Ladies Home Journal*, Mar. 1923, 16-17, and Florenz Ziegfeld Jr., "Showman's Shifting Sands," *Ladies Home Journal*, June 1923, 23.

19. Jeanne Thomas Allen discusses this in "The Film Viewer as Consumer," *Quarterly Review of Film Studies* 5, 4 (1980): 481-99. Lillian Russell was supplied gowns by Macy's as early as 1893, Allen points out, and she "was presented as an exponent of the proper behavior for women, and as a model of femininity" (487).

20. Stone, "The Ziegfeld Follies," 158. I am indebted to Stone's chapter 3, "Follies Opulence," 145-277, which provides details of costume and decor in these shows.

21. See Ann K. Clark, "The Girl: A Rhetoric of Desire," *Cultural Studies* 1, 2 (1987): 201, 200. Clark describes the familiar corporate image of The (usually blonde) Girl who is perpetually youthful and infinitely free, magical and sparkling. Clark's topic is The Girl as realized in late-twentieth-century corporate culture, but the resemblances to the rhetoric of the Ziegfeld Girl are striking.

22. Baral, *Revue*, 61. Cohen-Stratyner, "Welcome to 'Laceland,' " 317-18; see also her descriptions of the Ziegfeld Walk in "The Dance Direction of Ned Wayburn," 22-23, 150-52.

23. See Craik, *The Face of Fashion*, 56.

24. Cantor and Freedman, *Ziegfeld, the Great Glorifier*, 63.

25. Craik, *The Face of Fashion*, 70. For another discussion of the relationships between fashion and the body, see Elizabeth Wilson, "Fashion and the Postmodern Body," in *Chic Thrills: A Fashion Reader*, ed. Juliet Ash and Elizabeth Wilson (Berkeley: University of California Press, 1992), 3-16. See also Angela

Partington's discussion of gendered consumption in "Popular Fashion and Working-Class Affluence," 145–61, in the same volume.

26. Photos of the slenderness pledge are available at the Ziegfeld Archive, Harry Ransom Humanities Research Center, University of Texas at Austin. Photos of the "Curves" pledge can be found in the Hazel Forbes Photo File B, BRTC.

27. Diane Spaeter, "Ziegfeld Girls Recall the Fun of the Follies," *Los Angeles Evening Outlook* 16 June 1981.

28. "Ziegfeld's Secretary, a Puritan at Heart, Taught Showgirls How to Avoid Scandal," *Pittsburgh Press*, 5 Mar. 1937; and Judy Klemesrud, "Ziegfeld Girls—Recalling the Glitter of an Era," *New York Times*, 25 Apr. 1975.

29. Leslie W. Rabine, "A Woman's Two Bodies: Fashion Magazines, Consumerism, and Feminism," in *On Fashion*, ed. Shari Benstock and Suzanne Ferriss (New Brunswick, N.J.: Rutgers University Press, 1994), 59–75.

30. Bowlby, *Just Looking*, 32. Feminist film theorists have been especially interested in the overlapping appeals of the cinema screen and shop window in constituting the female spectator/consumer, and their debates are relevant to the female Ziegfeld audience member as well. See Gaylyn Studlar, "The Perils of Pleasure? Fan Magazine Discourse as Women's Commodified Culture in the 1920s," *Wide Angle* 13, 1 (1991): 6–33, and Miriam Hansen, "Adventures of Goldilocks: Spectatorship, Consumerism, and Public Life," *Camera Obscura* 22 (1990): 51–71.

31. Klemesrud, "Ziegfeld Girls—Recalling the Glitter of an Era."

32. "Ziegfeld Trade-Mark Asset to Chorus Girl," and Florenz Ziegfeld Jr.,"What Becomes of the Ziegfeld Follies Girls?" *Pictorial Review*, May 1925, 13.

33. Leach provides these details in *Land of Desire*, 67.

34. William R. Leach, "Transformations in a Culture of Consumption: Women and Department Stores, 1890–1925," *Journal of American History* 71, 2 (1984): 329–30. See also his descriptions of these particular retail events on 327 and 322. Susan Porter Benson points out the class dynamic of department stores in *Counter Cultures*, 77–78, 101–2.

35. Judith Williamson, "Woman Is an Island: Femininity and Colonization," in *Studies in Entertainment: Critical Approaches to Mass Culture*, ed. Tania Modleski (Bloomington: Indiana University Press, 1986), 115. Also see Laura E. Donaldson on the uses of colonial fantasy in marketing in *Decolonizing Feminisms: Race, Gender, and Empire-Building* (Chapel Hill: University of North Carolina Press, 1992), 88–89. Edward Said has reminded us that the Orient in particular has been characterized by the West as a different, more liberal, and desirable sexuality. See *Orientalism* (New York: Vintage, 1979).

36. Leach, "Transformations in a Culture of Consumption," 325.

37. "Florenz Ziegfeld," *Columbus Dispatch*, 16 July 1916, and "Picks 75 Chorus Girls from 3000 Aspirants," *Boston Herald*, 11 Apr. 1914.

38. See Toll, *On with the Show*, 243.

39. "This Is Julian Eltinge," *American Magazine*, May 1918: 36–37.

40. For the middle-class audience, Marybeth Hamilton points out, the female

illusionists were magicians, "able to conjure themselves across gender boundaries that all observers believed to be fixed and immutable." See " 'I'm the
Queen of the Bitches': Female Impersonation and Mae West's *Pleasure Man*,"
in *Crossing the Stage: Controversies on Cross-Dressing*, ed. Lesley Ferris (London:
Routledge, 1993), 111.

41. See, for example, Rennold Wolf, "The Sort of Fellow Julian Eltinge Really Is,"
Green Book, Nov. 1913, 793–803.

42. Historians Rapp and Ross make this point in "The Twenties' Backlash." In
the move to "restructure the family as a consumption unit," they point out,
female consumership was directly related to heterosexual desirability through
the double glamorization of female body and domestic products (93).

43. Garber, *Vested Interests*, 131–34.

44. Ibid., 17, 277.

4. Racialized, Glorified American Girls

1. Florenz Ziegfeld Jr., "Picking Out Pretty Girls for the Stage," 34+. Further
page references will be given parenthetically in the text. This article is reprinted in Roderick Nash, ed., *Call of the Wild: 1900–1916* (New York: Braziller,
1971), and quoted in Robert C. Allen, *Horrible Prettiness*, 272, and in Erenberg,
Steppin' Out, 219.

2. Doyle, *Bordering on the Body*, 41.

3. Florenz Ziegfeld Jr., "What Becomes of the Ziegfeld Follies Girls?" 12–13+.

4. Quoted in Ziegfeld's obituary, "Florenz Ziegfeld Dies in Hollywood after
Long Illness," *New York Times*, 23 July 1932.

5. See Florenz Ziegfeld Jr., "How I Pick Beauties," *Theatre Magazine*, Sept. 1919,
158–60, and Florenz Ziegfeld Jr., "How I Pick My Beauties," *Green Book*, Feb.
1914, 212–18.

6. "Picks 75 Chorus Girls from 3000 Aspirants," *Boston Herald*, 11 Apr. 1914;
"Chorus Girls Swarm, 1000 Answer Call from Ziegfeld," *New York Times*, 1 July
1927; "When Is a Woman's Figure Beautiful? Florenz Ziegfeld Tells How He
Judges," *New York Evening World*, 26 Dec. 1922.

7. Wolf, "The P. T. Barnum of the Theatre," 943.

8. "Stupendous Personality Contest: Florenz Ziegfeld Jr. Speaks on the Contest," *Movie Weekly*, 5 Aug. 1922.

9. See "When Is a Woman's Figure Beautiful?" and "Your Beauty May Be Made
or Marred Just by the Way You Wear Your Hair: Florenz Ziegfeld Jr. Explains
Why a Brunette Disposition and a Blonde Coiffure Are Sure to Make Trouble
for Their Owner," *New York Evening World*, 2 Jan. 1923.

10. "How Pretty Is a *Follies* Girl? Evelyn Law of the *Ziegfeld Follies* Has Perfect
Facial Measurements," *Picture Play*, May 1923, 47.

11. "Picks 75 Chorus Girls From 3000 Aspirants," and Florenz Ziegfeld Jr., "How
I Pick My Beauties."

12. See John Higham's extensive account of racism in regard to the nativist move-

ment in *Strangers in the Land: Patterns of American Nativism, 1860–1925* (New Brunswick, N.J.: Rutgers University Press, 1955), 131–57.

13. Florenz Ziegfeld Jr., "How I Pick Beauties," 160.

14. For further details on immigration during this era, see Thomas J. Archdeacon, *Becoming American: An Ethnic History* (New York: Free Press, 1983), 112–71.

15. See Banta's introduction to *Imaging American Women,* in which she argues that between 1876 and 1918, "Image-making and image-reading had become a major cultural activity, as well as the means for interpreting the nation's achievements and gauging its weaknesses. Even more, 'Woman' and 'American' coalesced around the types of desire and fear that underlay the very formation of that culture" (xxviii–xxix). The Ziegfeld article "Picking Out Pretty Girls for the Stage" illustrates why the Ziegfeld enterprise is an important case study of what Banta describes as a much larger social discourse.

16. "Beauty Contest Winner," *New York World,* 7 July 1907.

17. Banta, *Imaging American Women,* 112–13.

18. See Salvatore Cucchiari, "The Gender Revolution and the Transition from Bisexual Horde to Patrilocal Band: The Origins of Gender Hierarchy," in *Sexual Meanings: The Cultural Construction of Gender and Sexuality,* ed. Sherry B. Ortner and Harriet Whitehead (Cambridge: Cambridge University Press, 1981), 31–79, especially his discussion of racial and gender categories, 52–54.

19. H. H. Laughlin, quoted in Germaine Greer, *Sex and Destiny: The Politics of Human Fertility* (New York: Harper and Row, 1984), 313.

20. IQ differences between "native and immigrant stock" are cited in William Monroe Balch, "Is the Race Going Downhill?" *American Mercury,* Aug. 1926, 432–33. See also Albert Edward Wiggam, "The Rising Tide of Degeneracy: What Everybody Ought to Know about Eugenics," *World's Work,* Nov. 1926, 25–33, especially the immigration argument and the link to poetry, 30.

21. S. J. Holmes and J. C. Goff, "The Selective Elimination of Male Infants under Different Environmental Influences," and Frederick L. Hoffman, "The Problem of Negro-White Intermixture and Intermarriage," in *Eugenics in Race and State: Scientific Papers of the Second International Congress of Eugenics* (Baltimore: Williams and Wilkins, 1923), 2:233–51 and 2:175–88, respectively.

22. Madison Grant, *The Passing of the Great Race, or The Racial Basis of European History* (New York: Scribner's, 1916), 45. Further page references are given parenthetically in the text.

23. George F. Hall, *A Study in Bloomers, or The Model New Woman* (Chicago: American Bible House, 1895), 196.

24. Florence Guertin Tuttle, *The Awakening of Woman: The Psychic Side of Feminism* (New York: Abington, 1915), 126, 144.

25. Foucault, *The History of Sexuality: An Introduction,* 125.

26. Percy Hammond, "Women and Song (Ziegfeld Follies, 1917)," in *The Passionate Playgoer: A Personal Scrapbook,* ed. George Oppenheimer (New York: Viking, 1958), 554.

27. Kenneth R. Manning, "Race, Science, and Identity," in *Lure and Loathing: Essays on Race, Identity, and the Ambivalance of Assimilation*, ed. Gerald Early (New York: Penguin, 1993), 330, 325.

28. For details of Williams's public reception and the controversy of his appearance on the white stage, see Eric Ledell Smith, *Bert Williams: A Biography of the Pioneer Black Comedian* (Jefferson, N.C.: McFarland, 1992), 138–44 and 147–49.

29. The previous musical with an interracial cast, Will Marion Cook's *The Southerners*, 1904, had come from African American theater.

30. For an excellent description of the original stage production, see Miles Kreuger, *Show Boat: The Story of a Classic American Musical* (New York: Oxford University Press, 1977), 18–75. Kreuger also documents the changes in the 1929 film version; see pages 76–98.

31. Henry Louis Gates Jr., "The Welcome Table," in *Lure and Loathing*, ed. Early, 152.

32. "Dahomey on Broadway," *New York Times*, 19 Feb. 1903.

33. See Kathy Peiss, "Making Faces: The Cosmetics Industry and the Cultural Construction of Gender, 1890–1930," *Genders* 7 (1990): 143–69. Peiss points out that the industry was structured by clear social assumptions "linking whiteness with social success and refinement" (160).

34. Grant, *The Passing of the Great Race*, 16.

35. " 'Black and Tan' Drive Urged by Justices," *Variety*, 5 May 1926.

36. Quoted in Allen Woll, *Black Musical Theatre: From Coontown to Dream Girls* (1989; reprint, New York: De Capo, 1991), 109.

37. Ann Douglas, *Terrible Honesty: Mongrel Manhattan in the 1920s* (New York: Farrar, Straus, and Giroux 1995), 76.

38. See K. Sue Jewell, *From Mammy to Miss America and Beyond: Cultural Images and the Shaping of U.S. Social Policy* (London: Routledge, 1993), 37.

39. See Sander L. Gilman, "Black Bodies, White Bodies: Toward an Iconography of Female Sexuality in Late-Nineteenth-Century Art, Medicine, and Literature," in *"Race," Writing, and Difference*, ed. Henry Louis Gates Jr. (Chicago: University of Chicago Press, 1986), 223–61.

40. Lawrence W. Levine, *Highbrow/Lowbrow: The Emergence of Cultural Hierarchy in America* (Cambridge: Harvard University Press, 1988), 222.

41. Gilbert Seldes, "The Darktown Strutters on Broadway" (1922), in *The Seven Lively Arts* (1924; reprint, New York: A. S. Barnes, 1962), 147, 148–49.

42. "It's Getting Dark on Old Broadway," Louis A. Hirsch, Gene Buck, and Dave Stamper, 1922. See Woll, *Black Musical Theatre*, 51, 56, 76–77, 79. See also Douglas's account of the growing popularity of black music and entertainment in *Terrible Honesty*, 354–86.

43. Gilbert Seldes, "A Tribute to Florenz Ziegfeld" (1924), in *The Seven Lively Arts*, 141.

44. Lott, *Love and Theft*, 149.

45. Ibid., 4.

46. See Edward LeRoy Rice, *Monarchs of Minstrelsy from "Daddy" Rice to Date* (New York: Kenny, 1911), 179, 334, 354, 355.

47. "Miss Ginger of Jamaica," 1907, words and music by Billy Gaston, Ziegfeld Archive, Harry Ransom Humanities Research Center, University of Texas at Austin. Rosaline Stone points out the amorous slang meaning of the lyrics in "The Ziegfeld Follies," 38 n. 29.

48. Stone, "The Ziegfeld Follies," 83.

49. Douglas claims the Eastern and Mediterranean origins of Jewish music produced rhythms and keys compatible with African American music. See *Terrible Honesty*, 358.

50. Nancy Caldwell Sorel, "First Encounters: Fanny Brice and Florenz Ziegfeld," *Atlantic Monthly*, Jan. 1986, 81.

51. See Sophie Tucker, *Some of These Days* (New York: Doubleday, 1945), 33–35. For a contextualization of Tucker's sexual style, see Erenberg, *Steppin' Out*, 192–94.

52. As Pamela Brown points out in "Coon Shouting and the Americanization of the Jewish Ziegfeld Girl," the coon song's "red-hot mama" style conflates white sexuality with the sexuality of black mammy characters, masking yet another ethnicity of Jewish mother.

53. Barbara W. Grossman, *Funny Woman: The Life and Times of Fanny Brice* (Bloomington: Indiana University Press, 1991), 29–30.

54. Bert A. Williams, "The Negro on Stage," quoted by Smith, *Bert Williams*, 146.

55. See Ann Charters, *Nobody: The Story of Bert Williams* (London: Macmillan, 1970), 115. For the later conjectures on the contract, see Smith, *Bert Williams*, 132, and Mast, *Can't Help Singin'*, 22.

56. Grossman, *Funny Woman*, 43–44; Herbert G. Goldman, *Fanny Brice: The Original Funny Girl* (New York: Oxford University Press, 1992), 42. See also Goldman on the backstage and offstage prejudice against Bert Williams, 44.

57. "Girls from the 'Follies' Who've Made Good on the Screen," *Motion Picture Story*, Feb. 1932, 30.

58. Edmund Wilson, "The Finale at the Follies," *New Republic*, 25 Mar. 1925, 126.

59. Ibid., 125.

5. The Ziegfeld Girl and Hollywood Cinema

1. "Ziegfeld of the 'Follies' and the Way in Which He Glorifies the American Girl," *New York Evening Post*, 13 June 1925.

2. Bordman, *American Musical Revue*, 47–48. For another account of the decline of the revue and the transition to film, see Rubin, *Showstoppers*, 25–26, 30–32.

3. Mast, *Can't Help Singin'*, 117.

4. See Lucy Fischer's extended description of this dynamic in "The Image of Woman as Image: Optical Politics of *Dames*," in *Sexual Stratagems: The World of Women in Film*, ed. Patricia Erens (New York: Horizon, 1979), 41–61.

5. See Mast's description of the Berkeley-Ziegfeld continuum in *Can't Help Singin'*, 116–39. See also William D. Routt and Richard J. Thompson, " 'Keep Young and Beautiful': Surplus and Subversion in *Roman Scandals*," *Journal of Film and Video* 42, 1 (1990): 17–35. Routt and Thompson read the cinematic showgirl as a sign of performance (as opposed to talent) directly related to the *Ziegfeld Follies* and its arrangement of talented show business personalities versus the women "employed to stand and to move, to wear clothes, dressed and directed by men" (27).

6. See Rubin, *Showstoppers*, particularly chaps. 1–4. Rubin's focus is the continuum of Berkeley's work in theater and cinema, which Rubin sees as a specific example of the larger "tradition of spectacle" and its impact on the film musical. Rubin reads Berkeley through P. T. Barnum and Ziegfeld, persuasively illustrating the importance of theater history in cultural studies of cinema.

7. See Constance Balides's descriptions of such early films in "Scenarios of Exposure in the Practice of Everyday Life," and Robert C. Allen on the "smoking concert" film in *Horrible Prettiness*, 265–71.

8. "Fox in Talkies Only," *New York Times*, 25 Mar. 1929.

9. For the significance and influence of this film, see Richard Barrios, *A Song in the Dark: The Birth of the Musical Film* (New York: Oxford University Press, 1995), 59–76.

10. Richard Ziegfeld and Paulette Ziegfeld, *The Ziegfeld Touch*, 98.

11. Carter, *Ziegfeld: The Time of His Life*, 152. Rick Altman also emphasizes the significance of Ziegfeld, especially in the backstage musical film: "More than any other showman, Ziegfeld is responsible for the show musical's tendency to de-emphasize individual talent and to concentrate interest on the visual patterning of costumes and bodies." As a result, women dancers were "hoofers" rather than equal dance partners, a gender pattern Altman says is not limited to Busby Berkeley but is evident "throughout the entire show musical tradition." See *The American Film Musical*, 204.

12. The implications of the Queenie-Hank semiotics may have been displaced onto the blatant representations of male homosexuality in this film. In *A Song in the Dark*, Richard Barrios claims Zanfield's obviously gay costume designer is "the talkies' first gay stereotype" (75). Two other male backstage characters in this film are also teased sarcastically by more traditionally masculine characters; presumably, the film addresses audience knowledge about a gay male subculture active in the New York theater scene.

13. See Janet Staiger, *Interpreting Films: Studies in the Historical Reception of American Cinema* (Princeton: Princeton University Press, 1992), especially chap. 4, "Toward a Historical Materialist Approach to Reception Studies," 79–97. Following Staiger, my argument here is that "context-activated" studies can helpfully map out links between the film text and contextual discourses by assuming audiences use those other discourses as reading strategies.

14. Richard Dyer remarks that "women's only capital is their bodies as objects" in these depression musicals. See "Entertainment and Utopia," in *Genre: The Musical*, ed. Rick Altman (London: Routledge and Kegan Paul, 1981), 186.

15. Paris, *Louise Brooks*, 96.

16. "Girls from the 'Follies' Who've Made Good on the Screen," *Motion Picture Story*, Feb. 1932, 30.

17. Warren G. Harris, *The Other Marilyn: A Biography of Marilyn Miller* (New York: Arbor House, 1985).

18. "Reflections and News of the Screen World," *New York Times*, 27 July 1930.

19. "Juniors Act in New Film of Wolheim," *New York Times*, 27 Jan. 1929. Publicist Bernard Sobel recalls Ziegfeld's anti-Hollywood ad in "This Was Ziegfeld," 101.

20. Barrios, *A Song in the Dark*, 194. See Barrios's detailed description of this film on 194–98.

21. Charles Affron, "Performing Performing: Irony and Affect," *Cinema Journal* 20, 1 (1980): 44.

22. Rubin, *Showstoppers*, 89–90.

23. Mast, *Can't Help Singin'*, 119.

24. See Michael Rogin's excellent discussion of this film in "Making America Home: Racial Masquerade and Ethnic Assimilation in the Transition to Talking Pictures," *Journal of American History* 79 (1992): 1050–77. See also Henry Jenkins III, "Shall We Make It for New York or for Distribution? Eddie Cantor, *Whoopee*, and Regional Resistance to the Talkies," *Cinema Journal* 29, 3 (1990): 32–52.

25. Rogin, "Making America Home," 1076.

26. See Richard Ziegfeld and Paulette Ziegfeld, *The Ziegfeld Touch*, 170–71, for details of his final financial debacles.

27. Gilbert W. Gabriel, "Ziegfeld 'Ambition Artist to End,'" *New York American*, 24 July 1932; "A Master of Spectacle," *New York Times*, 25 July 1932.

28. See deCordova, *Picture Personalities*, 140. Raymond Williams explains his concept of "structure of feeling" in *The English Novel from Dickens to Lawrence* (London: Hogarth, 1984), 54. See also "Ziegfeld of the 'Follies' and the Way in Which He Glorifies the American Girl," *New York Evening Post*, 13 June 1925.

29. Wolf, "The P. T. Barnum of the Theatre."

30. "Brief Glimpse of Ziegfeld at Work," *New York Evening Journal*, 9 July 1917; Zoe Beckley, "On Laughs, Girls, and Dresses Ziegfeld Hunts For," *New York Evening Mail*, 13 June 1914; and Leander Richardson, "Monday Morning Interview," *New York Telegraph*, 19 June 1916.

31. "Picks 75 Chorus Girls from 3000 Aspirants."

32. Walter Tittle, "Ziegfeld of the Follies," *World's Work*, May 1927, 562–68.

33. Billie Burke correspondence, 15 Jan. 1923, Anna Held Museum Papers, BRTC.

34. "Ziegfeld First to Phone London," *New York Telegraph*, 8 Jan. 1927.

35. Cantor and Freedman, *Ziegfeld, the Great Glorifier*, 9, 14.

36. "Ziegfeld of the Follies and the Way in Which He Glorifies the American Girl," and Florenz Ziegfeld Jr., "What Becomes of the Ziegfeld Follies Girls?," 12.

37. "New Edition of Ziegfeld Follies Now in the Making," *New York American,* 13 June 1915.

38. Altman, *The American Film Musical,* 234.

39. F. Scott Fitzgerald, *The Great Gatsby* (1925; reprint, New York: Scribner's, 1953), 112.

40. Ibid., 41, 61.

41. "Follies Open on New York Roof," *New York American,* 27 June 1911. See also, for example, "Fifteenth Edition of Follies at the Globe, *New York American,* 22 June 1921, and "They All Turned Out for 'Follies,'" *New York Evening Graphic,* 2 July 1931.

42. See Robert Carringer, "*Citizen Kane, The Great Gatsby,* and Some Conventions of American Narrative," *Critical Inquiry* 2 (1975): 307–25.

43. See George F. Custen, *Bio/Pics: How Hollywood Constructed Public History* (New Brunswick, N.J.: Rutgers University Press, 1992), 18.

44. "Brief Glimpse of Ziegfeld at Work."

45. See J. C. Flugel, *The Psychology of Clothes* (1930; reprint, London: Hogarth, 1950), 118. Kaja Silverman has addressed the issue of the male fashion photographer or "connoisseur" of women in Lacanian terms as a form of disavowal of the need to be seen by the gaze of the Other. "It requires the male subject to see himself (and thus be seen) as 'the man who looks at women.'" See "Fragments of a Fashionable Discourse," in *Studies in Entertainment: Critical Approaches to Mass Culture,* ed. Tania Modleski (Bloomington: Indiana University Press, 1986), 143.

46. See deCordova, *Picture Personalities,* 118. See also "Ziegfeld Cables Denial of Charges," *New York Times,* 24 July 1922.

47. Cantor and Freedman, *Ziegfeld, the Great Glorifier,* 69.

48. Custen, *Bio/Pics,* 166.

49. Patricia Mellencamp, "The Sexual Economics of Gold Diggers of 1933," in *Close Viewings: An Anthology of New Film Criticism,* ed. Peter Lehman (Tallahassee: Florida State University Press, 1990), 191.

50. Harris, *The Other Marilyn,* 228.

51. Custen, *Bio/Pics,* 153.

52. Altman discusses the importance of this film as an MGM vehicle that acknowledged Busby Berkeley's work at Warner Brothers and set it up as the model for future musicals. See *The American Film Musical,* 234.

53. Cantor and Freedman, *Ziegfeld, the Great Glorifier,* 7–8.

54. Altman describes this development in the musical and points out that *Ziegfeld Girl* was one of the earliest to go this route, "foregrounding and undercutting the conventions of show musical syntax only in order to reaffirm them all the more convincingly" (ibid., 252). See also Altman's descriptions of the rise-to-stardom narrative in the musical on 226–34.

55. My reference here is Jane Feuer's well-known formulation in "The Self-Reflective Musical and the Myth of Entertainment," *Quarterly Review of Film Studies* 2, 3 (1977): 313–26. Feuer describes the alternation between exposure and mystification that ultimately works to reaffirm the "myths of entertainment."

56. See Richard Dyer's descriptions of how the story lines and characters "are tailored" for Garland, Lamarr, and Turner in "Lana: Four Films of Lana Turner," *Movie* 25 (1978): 30–52. See also Charles Affron's analysis of Lana Turner in this film in "Performing Performing." Affron points out Turner's disruptive effect in this film, "her need to be seen and desired by men as a movie star, as a Ziegfeld Girl, as a character within the fiction of the film" (46).

57. As Dyer writes, "In the big production numbers, it seems that the film does not quite know what to do with [Garland]." He draws attention especially to her costume in the "Minnie from Trinidad" number, granting that even though all the costumes are ridiculous, her goofy hat and the conflicting lines of her dress make clear that "she does not have and cannot carry off glamour." See *Heavenly Bodies*, 166–67.

58. Mast points out that in this film Ziegfeld is "a mere off-frame spirit, like God himself, represented in mortal affairs by his pope, Noble Sage (Edward Everett Horton)." See *Can't Help Singin'*, 117.

59. See Dyer's descriptions of these "walk-downs," which he reads as linking Sheila's moral decline specifically with the Ziegfeld show's signature female spectacle, implicating the entire Ziegfeld enterprise, in "Lana," 33–34.

60. See Dyer's extensive discussion of Garland's appeal to gay men, partially because of this status as not glamorous, in *Heavenly Bodies*, 141–94.

61. Julie Dash's 1982 independent film *Illusions* comments richly and ironically on this simultaneous black absence on-screen and the behind-the-scenes usage of black voices and music.

62. Mast traces this tension from Al Jolson's blackface in *The Jazz Singer* to the 1949 *Jolson Sings Again* in *Can't Help Singin'*, 89.

63. In the larger social scene, as bell hooks points out, "most white people do not have to 'see' black people (constantly appearing on billboards, television, movies, in magazines, etc.)" so that "they can live as though black people are invisible." See "Representing Whiteness in the Black Imagination," in *Cultural Studies*, ed. Lawrence Grossberg et al. (New York: Routledge, 1992), 340.

64. This taboo illustrates how race inflects codes of cinematic spectatorship and how female sexual display operates within specific "looking structures" involving both gender and race. See Jane Gaines, "White Privilege and Looking Relations: Race and Gender in Feminist Film Theory," in *Issues in Feminist Film Criticism*, ed. Patricia Erens (Bloomington: Indiana University Press, 1990), 197–214. For a history of the black showgirl and the limitations of Hollywood representation, see Donald Bogle, *Brown Sugar: Eighty Years of America's Black Female Superstars* (New York: Harmony, 1980).

65. Mast, *Can't Help Singin'*, 134.

66. These details come from Cohen, "The Dance Direction of Ned Wayburn," 161–62.

67. See Feuer on "the myth of spontaneity" in "The Self-Reflective Musical and the Myth of Entertainment." In addition, Chester's genius works in the tradition of depression musicals as described by Richard Hasbany: corporations are villainous and inhuman, but the individual genius entrepreneur is privileged and glamorized. See "The Musical Goes Ironic: The Evolution of Genres," *Journal of American Culture* 1 (1978): 128. On the capitalist ideology of depression era musicals, see Eric Smoodin, "Art/Work: Capitalism and Creativity in the Hollywood Musical," *New Orleans Review* 16, 1 (1989): 79–87.

68. See Siegfried Kracauer, "The Mass Ornament" (1927), trans. Barbara Correll and Jack Zipes, *New German Critique* 5 (1975): 67, on the mirroring effect of spectacle and spectator. See also J. P. Telotte, "A *Gold Digger* Aesthetic: The Depression Musical and its Audience," *Postscript* 1, 1 (1981): 18–24. Telotte describes the boundary-breaking effect of the typical Berkeley production number, "an illusion of a practically limitless, even labyrinthine world" (19).

69. Richard Dyer, "White," *Screen* 29, 4 (1988): 45, 47.

70. See Sharrar, *Avery Hopwood*, 114–19, for details of Hopwood's play and its circumstances. The wealthy marriages of Ziegfeld Girl Peggy Hopkins Joyce are described in David Grafton, "Peggy Hopkins Joyce, Inc.," *Forbes 400*, 23 Oct. 1989, 68–70.

71. See Rubin's descriptions of these numbers in *Showstoppers*, 103–6. Mellencamp has cited the influence of the Tiller Girls in the precision dancing, but I would add that the concepts of these numbers clearly recall the style of Berkeley's mentor, Ziegfeld. See "The Sexual Economics of *Gold Diggers of 1933*," 191.

72. Pamela Robertson sums up the major interpretations of this film in *Guilty Pleasures: Feminist Camp from Mae West to Madonna* (Durham: Duke University Press, 1996), 65–71, as well as offering her own feminist-camp reading of the narrative and production numbers on pages 57–65 and 70–73. Robertson's historicization of the gold digger and prostitute references in this film are especially helpful; see 74–84.

73. Ibid., 82. Robertson also points out that the Berkeley numbers are readable as lesbian enactments and eroticizations; see page 69.

74. For a description of the relationship between prostitution and theater in early American history, see Claudia D. Johnson, *American Actress: Perspective on the Nineteenth Century* (Chicago: Nelson-Hall, 1984), 13–16, 30. The association of chorus girls with prostitution is also discussed in Derek Parker and Julia Parker, *The Natural History of the Chorus Girl* (Indianapolis: Bobbs-Merrill, 1975), 11–14.

75. James Seymour, David Boehm, and Ben Markson, screenplay of *Gold Diggers of 1933*, in *Gold Diggers of 1933*, ed. Arthur Hove (Madison: University of Wisconsin Press, 1980), 54.

76. See Kathleen Rowe's analysis of this comic female figure in *The Unruly Woman: Gender and the Genres of Laughter* (Austin: University of Texas Press, 1995),

especially 25–49. Rowe lists androgyny as one of the signifiers of the unruly woman, but mixed gender signs can explicitly signify the lesbian as a more direct affront to heterosexuality.

77. Routt and Thompson claim the showgirl-money exchange is a " 'mad' riddle of value-meaning," because it is impossible to ascertain which party has received something more or less valuable, sexual pleasure or money: "Women receive what is really (culturally) of value in exchange for what is not. . . . But perhaps the men are receiving what is truly valuable and the women what is not." See " 'Keep Young and Beautiful,' " 27.

78. Mellencamp, "The Sexual Economics of *Gold Diggers of 1933*," 179.

79. *New York American,* 25 July 1932.

80. Quoted by Fred Lawrence Guiles, *Marion Davies* (New York: McGraw Hill, 1972), 65.

Epilogue: Showgirls

1. Marshall Sella, "Last Dance," *New York Times Magazine,* 17 Sept. 1995, 49. See also the Annie Leibovitz portfolio "Showgirls," *New Yorker,* 29 Jan. 1996, 69–77.

2. John Lahr, "My Mother the Ziegfeld Girl," *New Yorker,* 13 May 1996, 74–80.

3. See Barry Paris, "Profiles: The Godless Girl," *New Yorker,* 13 Feb. 1989, 54–73. See also Jeff Sewald, "Return of the Godless Girl," *American Film* 17 (1992): 14.

4. Lina Basquette, *Lina: DeMille's Godless Girl* (Fairfax, Va.: Denlinger's, 1990), 435.

5. Patricia J. Williams, *The Alchemy of Race and Rights: Diary of a Law Professor* (Cambridge: Harvard University Press, 1991), 116–17.

6. Robertson, *Guilty Pleasures,* 22.

7. See Moe Meyer's discussion of this effect in "Introduction: Reclaiming the Discourse of Camp," in *The Politics and Poetics of Camp,* ed. Meyer (London: Routledge, 1994), 10–11. This anthology makes the argument, summarized in Meyer's introduction, that camp is exclusively queer and/or gay or lesbian and that there is no nonqueer usage of camp except for derivation. The anthology's opening debate of camp as "style" or as queer critique seems to preclude that style itself can work as critique. For an argument enabling a more fluid constitution of camp and the queer, see Alisa Solomon, "It's Never Too Late to Switch," in *Crossing the Stage: Controversies on Cross-Dressing,* ed. Lesley Ferris (London: Routledge, 1993), 144–54.

8. Matthew Tinkcom describes this number as an example of Vincente Minnelli's camp sensibility and also of Garland's visual relationship to "the boys in the band" in some of her musicals. See "Working like a Homosexual: Camp Visual Codes and the Labor of Gay Subjects in the MGM Freed Unit," *Cinema Journal* 35, 2 (1996): 24–42.

9. In *Guilty Pleasures,* Robertson suggests that the camp, "alternative" reading of Garland may actually have been the dominant one—that is, that "women may have liked Garland for many of the same reasons as gay men" (62).

SELECT BIBLIOGRAPHY

Affron, Charles. "Performing Performing: Irony and Affect." *Cinema Journal* 20, 1 (1980): 42–52.

Allen, Jeanne Thomas. "The Film Viewer as Consumer." *Quarterly Review of Film Studies* 5, 4 (1980): 481–99.

Allen, Robert C. *Horrible Prettiness: Burlesque and American Culture.* Chapel Hill: University of North Carolina Press, 1991.

Allen, Theodore. *The Invention of the White Race.* London: Verso, 1994.

Althusser, Louis. "Ideology and Ideological State Apparatuses." In *Lenin and Philosophy, and Other Essays,* trans. Ben Brewster. New York: Monthly Review, 1971.

Altman, Rick. *The American Film Musical.* Bloomington: Indiana University Press, 1987.

Archdeacon, Thomas J. *Becoming American: An Ethnic History.* New York: Free Press, 1983.

Ash, Juliet, and Elizabeth Wilson, eds. *Chic Thrills: A Fashion Reader.* Berkeley: University of California Press, 1992.

Bailey, Peter. "Parasexuality and Glamour: The Victorian Barmaid as Cultural Prototype." *Gender and History* 2, 2 (1990): 148–72.

Balides, Constance. "Scenarios of Exposure in the Practice of Everyday Life: Women in the Cinema of Attractions." *Screen* 34, 1 (1993): 19–37.

Banner, Lois W. *American Beauty.* New York: Knopf, 1983.

Banta, Martha. *Imaging American Women: Idea and Ideals in Cultural History.* New York: Columbia University Press, 1987.

Baral, Robert. *Revue: A Nostalgic Reprise of the Great Broadway Period.* New York: Fleet, 1962.

Barber, Bernard, and Lyle S. Lobel. " 'Fashion' in Women's Clothes and the American Social System." *Social Forces* 31, 2 (1952): 124–31.

Barrios, Richard. *A Song in the Dark: The Birth of the Musical Film.* New York: Oxford University Press, 1995.

Basquette, Lina. *Lina: DeMille's Godless Girl.* Fairfax, Va.: Denlinger's, 1990.

Baty, S. Paige. *American Monroe: The Making of a Body Politic.* Berkeley and Los Angeles: University of California Press, 1995.

Benson, Susan Porter. *Counter Cultures: Saleswomen, Managers, and Customers in American Department Stores, 1890–1940.* Urbana: University of Illinois Press, 1986.

Benstock, Shari, and Suzanne Ferriss, eds. *On Fashion.* New Brunswick, N.J.: Rutgers University Press, 1994.

Bogle, Donald. *Brown Sugar: Eighty Years of America's Black Female Superstars.* New York: Harmony, 1980.

Bordman, Gerald. *American Musical Revue: From the Passing Show to Sugar Babies.* New York: Oxford University Press, 1985.

Bowlby, Rachel. *Just Looking: Consumer Culture in Dreiser, Gissing, and Zola*. New York: Methuen, 1985.

Braudy, Leo. *The Frenzy of Renown: Fame and Its History*. New York: Oxford University Press, 1986.

Burke, Billie. *With a Feather on My Nose*. New York: Appleton-Century-Crofts, 1949.

Cantor, Eddie, and David Freedman. *Ziegfeld, the Great Glorifier*. New York: Alfred H. King, 1934.

Carrera, Liane. *Anna Held and Flo Ziegfeld*. 1954. Trans. Guy Daniels. Hicksville, N.Y.: Exposition Press, 1979.

Carringer, Robert. "*Citizen Kane, The Great Gatsby,* and Some Conventions of American Narrative." *Critical Inquiry* 2 (1975): 307–25.

Carter, Randolph. *Ziegfeld: The Time of His Life*. 1974. Reprint, London: Bernard, 1988.

Castle, Terry. *The Apparitional Lesbian: Female Homosexuality and Modern Culture*. New York: Columbia University Press, 1993.

Charters, Ann. *Nobody: The Story of Bert Williams*. London: Macmillan, 1970.

Chauncey, George. *Gay New York: Gender, Urban Culture, and the Making of the Gay Male World, 1890–1940*. New York: Basic, 1994.

Clark, Ann K. "The Girl: A Rhetoric of Desire." *Cultural Studies* 1, 2 (1987): 200–207.

Cohen, Barbara Naomi. "The Dance Direction of Ned Wayburn: Selected Topics in Musical Staging, 1901–1923." Ph.D. diss., New York University, 1980.

Cohen-Stratyner, Barbara Naomi. "Welcome to 'Laceland': An Analysis of a Chorus Number from the Ziegfeld Follies of 1922, as Staged by Ned Wayburn." In Loney, *Musical Theatre in America*.

Craik, Jennifer. *The Face of Fashion: Cultural Studies in Fashion*. London: Routledge, 1994.

Cucchiari, Salvatore. "The Gender Revolution and the Transition from Bisexual Horde to Patrilocal Band: The Origins of Gender Hierarchy." In *Sexual Meanings: The Cultural Construction of Gender and Sexuality,* ed. Sherry B. Ortner and Harriet Whitehead. Cambridge: Cambridge University Press, 1981.

Curry, Ramona. *Too Much of a Good Thing: Mae West as Cultural Icon*. Minneapolis: University of Minnesota Press, 1996.

Curtin, Kaier. "*We Can Always Call Them Bulgarians*": *The Emergence of Lesbians and Gay Men on the American Stage*. Boston: Alyson, 1987.

Custen, George F. *Bio/Pics: How Hollywood Constructed Public History*. New Brunswick, N.J.: Rutgers University Press, 1992.

deCordova, Richard. *Picture Personalities: The Emergence of the Star System in America*. Urbana: University of Illinois Press, 1990.

de Lauretis, Teresa. *Technologies of Gender: Essays on Theory, Film, and Fiction*. Bloomington: Indiana University Press, 1987.

D'Emilio, John, and Estelle B. Freedman. *Intimate Matters: A History of Sexuality in America*. New York: Harper and Row, 1988.

Dijkstra, Bram. *Idols of Perversity: Fantasies of Feminine Evil in the Fin-de-Siècle Culture.* New York: Oxford University Press, 1986.

Donaldson, Laura E. *Decolonizing Feminisms: Race, Gender, and Empire-Building.* Chapel Hill: University of North Carolina Press, 1992.

Douglas, Ann. *Terrible Honesty: Mongrel Manhattan in the 1920s.* New York: Farrar, Straus, and Giroux, 1995.

Doyle, Laura. *Bordering on the Body: The Racial Matrix of Modern Fiction and Culture.* New York: Oxford University Press, 1994.

Duggan, Lisa. "The Social Enforcement of Heterosexuality and Lesbian Resistance in the 1920s." In Swerdlow and Lessinger, *Class, Race, and Sex.*

———. "The Trials of Alice Mitchell: Sensationalism, Sexology, and the Lesbian Subject in Turn-of-the-Century America. *Signs* 18, 4 (1993): 791–814.

Dyer, Richard. "Entertainment and Utopia." In *Genre: The Musical,* ed. Rick Altman. London: Routledge and Kegan Paul, 1981.

———. *Heavenly Bodies: Film Stars and Society.* New York: St. Martin's, 1986.

———. "Lana: Four Films of Lana Turner." *Movie* 25 (1978): 30–52.

———. "White." *Screen* 29, 4 (1988): 44–64.

———. *White.* London: Routledge, 1997.

Ellis, Havelock. *Studies in the Psychology of Sex: Sexual Inversion.* 1901. Reprint, Philadelphia: F. A. Davis, 1929.

Erenberg, Lewis A. *Steppin' Out: New York Nightlife and the Transformation of American Culture, 1890–1930.* 1981. Reprint, Chicago: University of Chicago Press, 1984.

Etherington-Smith, Meredith, and Jeremy Pilcher. *The "It" Girls: Lucy, Lady Duff Gordon, the Couturière "Lucile," and Elinor Glyn, Romantic Novelist.* San Diego: Harcourt Brace, 1986.

Faderman, Lillian. *Odd Girls and Twilight Lovers: A History of Lesbian Life in Twentieth-Century America.* New York: Penguin, 1991.

———. *Surpassing the Love of Men: Romantic Friendship and Love between Women from the Renaissance to the Present.* New York: Quill, 1981.

Farnsworth, Marjorie. *The Ziegfeld Follies: A History in Text and Pictures.* New York: Putnam's, 1956.

Ferris, Lesley, ed. *Crossing the Stage: Controversies on Cross-Dressing.* London: Routledge, 1993.

Feuer, Jane. "The Self-Reflective Musical and the Myth of Entertainment." *Quarterly Review of Film Studies* 2, 3 (1977): 313–26.

Finch, Casey. " 'Hooked and Buttoned Together': Victorian Underwear and Representations of the Female Body," *Victorian Studies* 34, 3 (1991): 337–63.

Fischer, Lucy. "The Image of Woman as Image: The Optical Politics of *Dames.*" In *Sexual Stratagems: The World of Women in Film,* ed. Patricia Erens. New York: Horizon, 1979.

Fitzgerald, F. Scott. *The Great Gatsby.* 1925. Reprint, New York: Scribner's, 1953.

Flugel, J. C. *The Psychology of Clothes.* 1930. Reprint, London: Hogarth, 1950.

Fordin, Hugh. *Getting to Know Him: A Biography of Oscar Hammerstein II.* New York: Random House, 1977.

Foucault, Michel. *The History of Sexuality.* 2 vols. Trans. Robert Hurley. 1978. Reprint, New York: Vintage, 1990.

Frankenberg, Ruth. *White Women, Race Matters: The Social Construction of Whiteness.* Minneapolis: University of Minnesota Press, 1993.

Friedberg, Anne. *Window Shopping: Cinema and the Postmodern.* Berkeley: University of California Press, 1993.

Gaines, Jane. "White Privilege and Looking Relations: Race and Gender in Feminist Film Theory." In *Issues in Feminist Film Criticism,* ed. Patricia Erens. Bloomington: Indiana University Press, 1990.

Gamson, Joshua. *Claims to Fame: Celebrity in Contemporary America.* Berkeley: University of California Press, 1994.

Garber, Marjorie. *Vested Interests: Cross-Dressing and Cultural Anxiety.* 1992. Reprint, New York: HarperPerennial, 1993.

Gates, Henry Louis, Jr. "The Welcome Table." In *Lure and Loathing: Essays on Race, Identity, and the Ambivalance of Assimilation,* ed. Gerald Early. New York: Penguin, 1993.

Gilfoyle, Timothy J. "Policing of Sexuality." In Taylor, *Inventing Times Square.*

Gilman, Sander L. "Black Bodies, White Bodies: Toward an Iconography of Female Sexuality in Late-Nineteenth-Century Art, Medicine, and Literature." In *"Race," Writing, and Difference,* ed. Henry Louis Gates Jr. Chicago: University of Chicago Press, 1986.

Glenn, Susan A. *Daughters of the Shtetl: Life and Labor in the Immigrant Generation.* Ithaca, N.Y.: Cornell University Press, 1990.

Goldman, Herbert G. *Fanny Brice: The Original Funny Girl.* New York: Oxford University Press, 1992.

Grafton, David. "Peggy Hopkins Joyce, Inc." *Forbes 400,* 23 Oct. 1989, 68–70.

Grant, Madison. *The Passing of the Great Race, or The Racial Basis of European History.* New York: Scribner's, 1916.

Greer, Germaine. *Sex and Destiny: The Politics of Human Fertility.* New York: Harper and Row, 1984.

Grossman, Barbara W. *Funny Woman: The Life and Times of Fanny Brice.* Bloomington: Indiana University Press, 1991.

Grosz, Elizabeth. *Volatile Bodies: Toward a Corporeal Feminism.* Bloomington: Indiana University Press, 1994.

Guiles, Fred Lawrence. *Marion Davies.* New York: McGraw Hill, 1972.

Hamilton, Marybeth. " 'I'm the Queen of the Bitches': Female Impersonation and Mae West's *Pleasure Man.*" In *Crossing the Stage: Controversies on Cross-Dressing,* ed. Lesley Ferris. London: Routledge, 1993.

Hammond, Percy. "Women and Song (Ziegfeld Follies, 1917)." In *The Passionate Playgoer: A Personal Scrapbook,* ed. George Oppenheimer. New York: Viking, 1958.

Hansen, Miriam. "Adventures of Goldilocks: Spectatorship, Consumerism, and Public Life." *Camera Obscura* 22 (1990): 51–71.

Harris, Warren G. *The Other Marilyn: A Biography of Marilyn Miller.* New York: Arbor House, 1985.

Hasbany, Richard. "The Musical Goes Ironic: The Evolution of Genres." *Journal of American Culture* 1 (1978): 120–37.

Higham, Charles. *Ziegfeld.* Chicago: Regnery, 1972.

Higham, John. *Strangers in the Land: Patterns of American Nativism, 1860–1925.* New Brunswick, N.J.: Rutgers University Press, 1955.

Hirsch, John. "The American Revue Costume." In Loney, *Musical Theatre in America.*

hooks, bell. "Representing Whiteness in the Black Imagination." In *Cultural Studies,* ed. Lawrence Grossberg et al. New York: Routledge, 1992.

Hove, Arthur, ed. *Gold Diggers of 1933.* Madison: University of Wisconsin Press, 1980.

International Congress of Eugenics. *Eugenics in Race and State: Scientific Papers of the Second International Congress of Eugenics.* 2 vols. Baltimore: Williams and Wilkins, 1923.

Jenkins, Henry, III. "Shall We Make It for New York or for Distribution? Eddie Cantor, *Whoopee,* and Regional Resistance to the Talkies." *Cinema Journal* 29, 3 (1990): 32–52.

Jewell, K. Sue. *From Mammy to Miss America and Beyond: Cultural Images and the Shaping of U.S. Social Policy.* London: Routledge, 1993.

Johnson, Claudia D. *American Actress: Perspective on the Nineteenth Century.* Chicago: Nelson-Hall, 1984.

Katz, Jonathan Ned. *The Invention of Heterosexuality.* New York: Dutton, 1995.

Kracauer, Siegfried. "The Mass Ornament." 1927. Trans. Barbara Correll and Jack Zipes. *New German Critique* 5 (1975): 67–76.

Krafft-Ebing, Richard von. *Psychopathia Sexualis.* 1906. Reprint, New York: Physicians and Surgeons Book Company, 1926.

Kreuger, Miles. *Show Boat: The Story of a Classic American Musical.* New York: Oxford University Press, 1977.

Kunzle, David. "Dress Reform as Antifeminism: A Response to Helene E. Robert's 'The Exquisite Slave: The Role of Clothing in the Making of the Victorian Woman,'" *Signs* 2, 3 (1977): 570–79.

Lahr, John. "My Mother the Ziegfeld Girl." *New Yorker,* 13 May 1996, 74–80.

Lasser, Michael. "The Glorifier: Florenz Ziegfeld and the Creation of the American Showgirl." *American Scholar* 63 (1994): 441–48.

Leach, William R. *Land of Desire: Merchants, Power, and the Rise of a New American Culture.* New York: Pantheon, 1993.

———. "Transformations in a Culture of Consumption: Women and Department Stores, 1890–1925" *Journal of American History* 71, 2 (1984): 319–42.

Leibovitz, Annie. "Showgirls." *New Yorker,* 29 January 1996, 69–77.

Lessard, Suzannah. "Stanford White's Ruins." *New Yorker,* 8 July 1996, 49–65.

Levine, Lawrence W. *Highbrow/Lowbrow: The Emergence of Cultural Hierarchy in America.* Cambridge: Harvard University Press, 1988.

Loney, Glenn, ed. *Musical Theatre in America*. Westport, Conn.: Greenwood, 1984.

Lott, Eric. *Love and Theft: Blackface Minstrelsy and the American Working Class*. New York: Oxford University Press, 1993.

Lubow, Arthur. *The Reporter Who Would Be King: A Biography of Richard Harding Davis*. New York: Scribner's, 1992.

McArthur, Benjamin. *Actors and American Culture, 1880–1920*. Philadelphia: Temple University Press, 1984.

McCardell, Roy L. *Conversations of a Chorus Girl*. New York: Street and Smith, 1903.

McEvoy, J. P. "He Knew What They Wanted." *Saturday Evening Post*, 10 Sept. 1932, 10+.

————. *Show Girl*. New York: Simon and Schuster, 1928.

Manning, Kenneth R. "Race, Science, and Identity." In *Lure and Loathing: Essays on Race, Identity, and the Ambivalance of Assimilation*, ed. Gerald Early. New York: Penguin, 1993.

Maschio, Geraldine A. "The Ziegfeld Follies: Form, Content, and the Significance of an American Revue." Ph.D. diss., University of Wisconsin Madison, 1981.

Mast, Gerald. *Can't Help Singin': The American Musical on Stage and Screen*. Woodstock, N.Y.: Overlook, 1987.

Mellencamp, Patricia. "The Sexual Economics of *Gold Diggers of 1933*." In *Close Viewings: An Anthology of New Film Criticism*, ed. Peter Lehman. Tallahassee: Florida State University Press, 1990.

Merton, Madge. *Confessions of a Chorus Girl*. New York: Grafton, 1903.

Meyer, Moe, ed. *The Politics and Poetics of Camp*. London: Routledge, 1994.

Mooney, Michael MacDonald. *Evelyn Nesbit and Stanford White: Love and Death in the Gilded Age*. New York: William Morrow, 1976.

Mulvey, Laura. "Visual Pleasure and Narrative Cinema." *Screen* 16 (1975): 6–18.

Nathan, George J. "Ziegfeld." 1923. Reprinted in *The Magic Mirror*. New York: Alfred A. Knopf, 1960.

Ohmann, Richard. "History and Literary History: The Case of Mass Culture." In *Modernity and Mass Culture*, ed. James Naremore and Patrick Brantlinger. Bloomington: Indiana University Press, 1991.

Paris, Barry. *Louise Brooks*. New York: Knopf, 1989.

————. "Profiles: The Godless Girl." *New Yorker*, 13 Feb. 1989, 54–73.

Parker, Derek, and Julia Parker. *The Natural History of the Chorus Girl*. Indianapolis: Bobbs-Merrill, 1975.

Partington, Angela. "Popular Fashion and Working-Class Affluence." In Ash and Wilson, *Chic Thrills*.

Peiss, Kathy. *Cheap Amusements: Working Women and Leisure in Turn-of-the-Century New York*. Philadelphia: Temple University Press, 1986.

————. "Making Faces: The Cosmetics Industry and the Cultural Construction of Gender, 1890–1930. *Genders* 7 (1990): 143–69.

Pollock, Channing. *Harvest of My Years: An Autobiography*. Indianapolis: Bobbs-Merrill, 1943.

Powers, John Robert. *The Powers Girls: The Story of Models and Modeling and the Natural Steps by Which Attractive Girls Are Created.* New York: E. P. Dutton, 1941.

Pumphrey, Martin. "The Flapper, the Housewife, and the Making of Modernity." *Cultural Studies* 1 (1987): 179–94.

Rabine, Leslie W. "A Woman's Two Bodies: Fashion Magazines, Consumerism, and Feminism." In Benstock and Ferriss, *On Fashion.*

Rapp, Rayna, and Ellen Ross. "The Twenties' Backlash: Compulsory Heterosexuality, the Consumer Family, and the Waning of Feminism." In Swerdlow and Lessinger, *Class, Race, and Sex.*

Rice, Edward LeRoy. *Monarchs of Minstrelsy from "Daddy" Rice to Date.* New York: Kenny, 1911.

Robertson, Pamela. *Guilty Pleasures: Feminist Camp from Mae West to Madonna.* Durham: Duke University Press, 1996.

Rogin, Michael. "Making America Home: Racial Masquerade and Ethnic Assimilation in the Transition to Talking Pictures." *Journal of American History* 79 (1992): 1050–77.

Rosenfeld, Lulla Adler. *The Yiddish Theatre and Jacob P. Adler.* 2d ed. New York: Shapolsky, 1988.

Routt, William D., and Richard J. Thompson. " 'Keep Young and Beautiful': Surplus and Subversion in *Roman Scandals." Journal of Film and Video* 42, 1 (1990): 17–35.

Rubin, Martin. *Showstoppers: Busby Berkeley and the Tradition of Spectacle.* New York: Columbia University Press, 1993.

Ryan, Mary P. *Womanhood in America: From Colonial Times to the Present.* New York: Franklin Watts, 1983.

Scott, Joan. *Gender and the Politics of History.* New York: Columbia University Press, 1988.

Seldes, Gilbert. "The Great Glorifier." *New Yorker,* 31 May 1993, 60–61. First published in *New Yorker,* July 25–Aug. 1, 1931, 18–22.

———. *The Seven Lively Arts.* 1924. Reprint, New York: A. S. Barnes, 1962.

Senelick, Laurence. "Private Parts in Public Places." In Taylor, *Inventing Times Square.*

Sewald, Jeff. "Return of the Godless Girl." *American Film* 17 (1992): 14.

Seymour, James, David Boehm, and Ben Markson. Screenplay of *Gold Diggers of 1933.* In Hove, *Gold Diggers of 1933.*

Sharrar, Jack F. *Avery Hopwood: His Life and Plays.* Jefferson, N.C.: McFarland, 1989.

Silverman, Kaja. "Fragments of a Fashionable Discourse." In *Studies in Entertainment: Critical Approaches to Mass Culture,* ed. Tania Modleski, 139–52. Bloomington: Indiana University Press, 1986.

Simmons, Christina. "Companionate Marriage and the Lesbian Threat." *Frontiers* 4, 3 (1979): 54–59.

———. "Modern Sexuality and the Myth of Victorian Repression." In *Passion and Power: Sexuality in History,* ed. Kathy Peiss and Christina Simmons. Philadelphia: Temple University Press, 1989.

Smith, Eric Ledell. *Bert Williams: A Biography of the Pioneer Black Comedian*. Jefferson, N.C.: McFarland, 1992.

Smith-Rosenberg, Carroll. *Disorderly Conduct: Visions of Gender in Victorian America*. New York: Knopf, 1985.

Smoodin, Eric. "Art/Work: Capitalism and Creativity in the Hollywood Musical." *New Orleans Review* 16, 1 (1989): 79–87.

Sobel, Bernard. "This Was Ziegfeld." *American Mercury*, Jan. 1945, 96–102.

Sorel, Nancy Caldwell. "First Encounters: Fanny Brice and Florenz Ziegfeld." *Atlantic Monthly*, Jan. 1986, 81.

Staiger, Janet. *Interpreting Films: Studies in the Historical Reception of American Cinema*. Princeton: Princeton University Press, 1992.

Stallybrass, Peter, and Allon White. *The Politics and Poetics of Transgression*. Ithaca, N.Y.: Cornell University Press, 1986.

Stanfield, Peter. " 'An Octoroon in the Kindling': American Vernacular and Blackface Minstrelsy in 1930s Hollywood." *Journal of American Studies* 31 (1997): 407–38.

Stone, Rosaline B. "The Ziegfeld Follies: A Study of Theatrical Opulence from 1907 to 1931." Ph.D. diss., University of Denver, 1985.

Strom, Sharon Hartman. *Beyond the Typewriter: Gender, Class, and the Origins of Modern American Office Work*. Urbana: University of Illinois Press, 1992.

Studlar, Gaylyn. "The Perils of Pleasure? Fan Magazine Discourse as Women's Commodified Culture in the 1920s." *Wide Angle* 13, 1 (1991): 6–33.

Swerdlow, Amy, and Hanna Lessinger, eds. *Class, Race, and Sex: The Dynamics of Control*. Boston: G. K. Hall, 1983.

Taylor, William R., ed. *Inventing Times Square: Commerce and Culture at the Crossroads of the World*. New York: Russell Sage, 1991.

Teitel, Nathan. "The Man Who Invented Women." *Saturday Review*, 4 Nov. 1972, 84–86.

Telotte, J. P. "A *Gold Digger* Aesthetic: The Depression Musical and Its Audience." *Postscript* 1, 1 (1981): 18–24.

Tinkcom, Matthew. "Working like a Homosexual: Camp Visual Codes and the Labor of Gay Subjects in the MGM Freed Unit." *Cinema Journal* 35, 2 (1996): 24–42.

Toll, Robert C. *On with the Show: The First Century of Show Business in America*. New York: Oxford University Press, 1976.

Tucker, Sophie. *Some of These Days*. New York: Doubleday, 1945.

Turim, Maureen. "Seduction and Elegance: The New Woman of Fashion in Silent Cinema." In Benstock and Ferriss, *On Fashion*.

Ware, Vron. *Beyond the Pale: White Women, Racism, and History*. London: Verso, 1992.

Weiss, Andrea. *Vampires and Violets: Lesbians in Film*. New York: Penguin, 1992.

Wertheim, Arthur Frank, ed. *Will Rogers at the Ziegfeld Follies*. Norman: University of Oklahoma Press, 1992.

Williams, Patricia J. *The Alchemy of Race and Rights: Diary of a Law Professor.* Cambridge: Harvard University Press, 1991.

Wilson, Edmund. "The Finale at the Follies." *New Republic,* 25 Mar. 1925, 125–26.

———. "The Follies as an Institution." 1923. Reprinted in *The Portable Edmund Wilson.* Ed. Lewis M. Dabney. New York: Viking, 1983.

Wilson, Elizabeth. "Fashion and the Postmodern Body." In Ash and Wilson, *Chic Thrills.*

Wodehouse, P. G., and Guy Bolton. *Bring On the Girls! The Improbable Story of Our Life in Musical Comedy.* New York: Simon and Schuster, 1953.

Wolf, Rennold. "The P. T. Barnum of the Theatre." *Green Book,* June 1914, 933–46.

———. "The Sort of Fellow Julian Eltinge Really Is." *Green Book,* Nov. 1913, 793–803.

Woll, Allen. *Black Musical Theatre: From Coontown to Dream Girls.* 1989. Reprint, New York: De Capo, 1991.

Woollcott, Alexander. "The Invisible Fish." In *The Portable Woollcott.* Ed. Joseph Hennessey. New York: Viking, 1946. First published in *Colliers,* 26 Oct. 1929.

Ziegfeld, Florenz, Jr., "Beauty, the Fashions, and the Follies." *Ladies Home Journal,* Mar. 1923, 16+.

———. "How I Pick Beauties." *Theatre Magazine,* Sept. 1919, 158–60.

———. "How I Pick My Beauties," *Green Book,* Feb. 1914, 212–18.

———. "Picking Out Pretty Girls for the Stage." *American Magazine,* Dec. 1919: 34+.

———. "Showman's Shifting Sands." *Ladies Home Journal,* June 1923, 23+.

———. "What Becomes of the Ziegfeld Follies Girls?" *Pictorial Review,* May 1925, 12–13+.

Ziegfeld, Patricia. *The Ziegfelds' Girl: Confessions of an Abnormally Happy Childhood.* Boston: Little, Brown, 1964.

Ziegfeld, Richard, and Paulette Ziegfeld. *The Ziegfeld Touch: The Life and Times of Florenz Ziegfeld, Jr.* New York: Abrams, 1993.

INDEX